The International Librai

THE MENTAL DEVELOPMENT
OF THE CHILD

Founded by C. K. Ogden

The International Library of Psychology

DEVELOPMENTAL PSYCHOLOGY
In 32 Volumes

THE MENTAL DEVELOPMENT OF THE CHILD

A Summary of Modern Psychological Theory

KARL BÜHLER

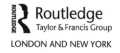
Routledge
Taylor & Francis Group

LONDON AND NEW YORK

First published in 1930 by
Routledge, Trench, Trubner & Co., Ltd.

Reprinted in 1999, 2000, 2002 by
Routledge
2 Park Square, Milton Park, Abingdon, Oxon, OX14 4RN
Simultaneously published in the USA and Canada by Routledge
711 Third Avenue, New York, NY 10017

Transferred to Digital Printing 2007

Routledge is an imprint of the Taylor & Francis Group, an informa business

First issued in paperback 2013

© 1930 Karl Bühler
Translated from the Fifth German Edition by Oscar Oeser

The publishers have made every effort to contact authors/copyright holders
of the works reprinted in the *International Library of Psychology*.
This has not been possible in every case, however, and we would
welcome correspondence from those individuals/companies
we have been unable to trace.

These reprints are taken from original copies of each book. In many cases
the condition of these originals is not perfect. The publisher has gone to
great lengths to ensure the quality of these reprints, but wishes to point
out that certain characteristics of the original copies will, of necessity, be
apparent in reprints thereof.

British Library Cataloguing in Publication Data
A CIP catalogue record for this book
is available from the British Library

The Mental Development of the Child

ISBN 978-0-415-20986-1 (hbk)
ISBN 978-0-415-86883-9 (pbk)

CONTENTS

CHAPTER ONE

CHAPTER TWO

Note :—It is now the general custom to write the age of children in years and months thus : 5 ; 3, that is, at the age of five years and three months, or more accurately, in the fourth month of the sixth year of life.

LIST OF ILLUSTRATIONS

PREFACE

THE German edition of this book first appeared in 1919, since when it has gone through five editions. It is intended for students and teachers, and is a short summary of the substance of my larger work, *Die geistige Entwicklung des Kindes.*

The study of childhood is to-day a rapidly advancing and intensively cultivated science, whose results can be presented from widely different points of view. In this book the concept of development is the central pivot. It is shown how progress is made in the chief forms of child activity—in speech and thinking, in play, drawings and social behaviour—from the primitive state of animals to those activities that distinguish man from the animals. The plan and theme is a study of the child's development in longitudinal section, as it were.

A complement to such a book has long been wanted in our science. It has at last been supplied by Charlotte Bühler who, to put it briefly, has studied this development in cross section. In her book, *Kindheit und Jugend* (1928), she has divided the whole drama of development into five periods, which are all causally interdependent. It is based on the researches carried out in Vienna. The reader is therefore referred to her book as a complement to this.

VIENNA,   KARL BÜHLER.
December, 1929.

THE
MENTAL DEVELOPMENT
OF THE CHILD

CHAPTER ONE

GENERAL CONSIDERATIONS

1.—INSTINCT, TRAINING, AND INTELLECT

A CHAPTER FROM COMPARATIVE PSYCHOLOGY

ONE can speak in different senses of the developmental course of the mind, but here we are thinking of what is reflected in the growing child : entering the world more helpless than most animals, entirely passive and as yet devoid of all mental activity, it stands before us, three years later, a thinking being that has far surpassed all animals. Very far surpassed, for it speaks a human language, passes judgments, draws conclusions, has some idea—however primitive and imperfect—of the world, and takes up a tentative attitude towards the true and the false, the good and the bad, the beautiful and the ugly. This *humanization* of the child constitutes our theme.

Occasionally, however, it will be profitable to extend the scope somewhat and to compare the development of the individual with the history of the species, with the history of mankind. The language and art, the conception of the world, the conduct of life of the older generation into which the child grows, once had their beginning too ; once there must have been an early and

an earliest ' childhood' of humanity in which human
language, drawing on clay and stone, music and plastic
art were developed ; and a still more remote time when
man first created tools.

We know very little about these primitive times and
yet a resigned " *ignorabimus* " would be premature ;
for the science of prehistory has not yet exhausted its
best source of information, nor yet indeed in many
respects succeeded in recognizing it.   This source, I feel
convinced, is the mental development of *our* children.
We are beginning to see, e.g., in the language and drawing
of children, certain fundamental laws of mental progress
manifesting themselves quite independently of external
influences, laws which, as they govern the evolution of
childhood, in like manner presumably governed that of
prehistory.   Whoever formulates them correctly will be
able to render very valuable service to prehistory, or
at least to put forward fruitful questions.   We shall
discuss details at a later stage.

But more important for our purposes is the ultimate
enlargement of our point of view : man is not isolated in
the world, but is related to the animals.   On examining
all significant, i.e. (objectively) purposeful modes of behaviour displayed by man and animals, we find a very
simple and obvious structure consisting of three great
stages in ascending order ;   these three stages are called
instinct, training and intellect.   As matters stand to-day,
instinct is the lowest stage and at the same time the soil
from which all the higher ones grow.   Even in man
there is no field or form of mental activity which is not
in some way based on the instincts.   It is true that in
former times, in the seventeenth and eighteenth centuries,
philosophers were a little too free with special terms.
The sociologist used to speak of a ' social instinct ' and
an ' instinct of property ' in man, the philologist of an
' instinct of communication ' and other students attributed
to man religious, ethical, æsthetic instincts.   It almost
seemed as if these thinkers imagined the new-born child

as an ambassador entering life with a bundle of complete programmes. It was only too easy to criticize so crude a conception of instinct, for human instincts are undoubtedly not so clearly defined and determined. But the underlying assumption that the highest forms of the mind, society, law, language, art and religion, are intimately dependent on instincts is not thereby refuted. But let us first endeavour to get our minds clear on the fundamental concepts.

(a) *What is instinct?* A chicken, as soon as it has left the shell, runs about, picks up grains, and drinks water after the fashion of fowls ; a duckling on the first day of its life swims and dives to perfection. No one has shown the animals how to do these things ; no useful or harmful experiences have gone before ; we call it instinctive behaviour. There are animals whose life consists entirely, or almost entirely, of such events, viz., the insects and other invertebrates. I shall take as a simple example the well-known ant-lions, larvæ of a certain group of neuroptera, because they have recently been subjected to a very thorough study.[1] At the bottom of a sandpit with steep sides, which it has dug itself, the tiny robber conceals himself, buried up to the head. With its strong, sharp-edged jaws it is not unlike a stag-beetle, though no bigger than a large ant. As soon as an ant or a little spider strays on to the edge of the pit and falls down its steep sides, the ant-lion's jaws close with a snap. If the victim is able to get a hold half-way up and starts to climb out, the danger is not past, for the ant-lion hurls grains of sand with great force against its victim and generally succeeds in bringing it down. Once it is caught, its blood is slowly sucked out. In a good, profitable hole of this kind the ant-lion will stay for months, i.e., during practically the whole of its larval existence. It is only when no victims arrive and hunger drives it, or when from other circumstances living conditions are

---

[1] Fr. Doflein, *Der Ameisenlöwe. Eine biologische, tierpsychologische und reflexbiologische Untersuchung.* Jena, 1916.

no longer favourable, that it leaves the pit and crawls towards light, warmth and dryness, until it has found a suitable new place where it again digs itself in. This is undoubtedly " sensible," i.e., purposive behaviour, and yet it consists, as Doflein has shown quite clearly, of a very small number of simple reflexes. In an experiment the animal behaves almost like an automaton. It is practically ready to begin as soon as it leaves the egg and alters little during its life. Once one knows the few factors in question, one can always say in any situation what will happen, and can produce any meaningless actions one desires. There are good reasons, nevertheless, for assuming that it is not a pure reflex-automaton ; but that is a different matter.

In such examples the properties of *pure* instinctive actions can be most readily observed : that from the beginning such acts are carried out with considerable perfection without previous practice, that they are cut out for certain conditions of life and these only, that they occur uniformly in all individuals of a species, etc., in short, that they are *a ready-for-use inheritance of modes of behaviour* set going in a definite way according to a preformed natural plan. It is true that matters are not everywhere so simple and obvious as in the case of the ant-lion ; among the instincts are found extraordinarily complicated activities of which it cannot be predicted what factors are at work until more exact experiments have been performed. Biology is at present hard at work trying to separate the simple factors from the complex ones. When once these are known as well as the constituent parts of the animal body, a very great deal will have been gained. But there are cases, particularly among the higher animals, where it is difficult, if not impossible, to say how much of a given performance is due to instinct and how much to training or, when the possibility of it arises at all, how much to intellect ; this overlapping is part of the problem and does not affect the validity of our conceptual distinction of three stages.

The psychologist is not at present able to say much about the instincts.[1] Whether there is something akin to a soul in them which governs and co-ordinates reflexes, whether the insects, e.g., have feeling and sensation at all and how they "feel" before, during and after an act, are all questions that cannot be answered offhand to-day. There is as much justification for the assumption that insects are richly endowed with desires, emotions, etc., as for the contrary assumption that their conscious life has not yet progressed anything like as far. I think we ought to hold only to the view that nature never makes superfluous provision, never gives consciousness where it can be dispensed with in a group without prejudicing its existence. Belief in a consciousness which, like the phenomenon of the day of rest, exists side by side with mechanical events without exerting any influence on them, flies in the face of all biological doctrine. Possibly, the most universal facts of organic being (growth, propagation, regeneration) demand the supposition of a *mind-like factor* in all life,[2] nevertheless the question as to the *functions of consciousness* is so obscure that, for the time being, we must leave it quite out of account in our doctrine of instincts.

This being so, we must simply content ourselves with looking at things from the outside. Instincts have an extremely conservative character; they function with extraordinary certainty and precision where everything remains unaltered, and fail when the individual enters upon new conditions of existence. Naturally they once had to come into being too, and were not exempt from change, but this only came about in the course of and at the cost of many generations.

(b) *Training.* Nature has accomplished marvellous things with instincts, but there were definite limits here, and further development has taken place along different

---

[1] Cf. my survey, "Die Instinkte des Menschen." ix. *Kongress für Experim. Psychol.* München, 1926.

[2] H. Driesch, *Die organischen Regulationen*, 1901; *Die "Seele" als elementarer Naturfaktor*, 1903, *Philosophie des Organischen*, 1909.

lines. The inflexibility of instinct was broken down more and more and the individual became capable of adapting himself to the special conditions of his environment, became capable of learning. The first step in this direction is called *associative memory*, or in other words, training. A young dog has the instinct to hunt, but by no means always sticks to one unchanging method in its hunting. The dog learns to exploit new possibilities, as every huntsman knows. In order to break an animal in properly, one starts off from the instincts it has already. So, e.g., a dog reacts by nature to traces of smell, pursues a living animal and brings back in its jaws the booty it has captured. It is with this capital of instinctive modes of behaviour that training works, *by suppressing some, accentuating others and forming new combinations.* When a setter gets near the hiding game, he has to keep still until the hunter has rustled it and brought it down. That is opposed to the dog's primitive method of hunting, and its desire to leap on to the hunted animal must be suppressed by training ; or if a certain breed of dog has inherited the acquired property of setting, this must be intensified by training. We can see that the dog's unwearying zeal for hunting is an enhancement, and that retrieving is a combination, of original modes of behaviour (carrying off the booty and returning to the master).

The human trainer deals in reward and punishment and thereby merely imitates what nature shows him, for in its wild state the animal also learns *by success and failure.* Take as an example the hen at the garden fence. At first she will run up and down restlessly in front of the obstacle until by chance she lights upon a suitable opening. The second, third, fifth time the hen behaves no differently, but when the same process is repeated a few dozen times, she gradually reaches the goal more quickly and eventually avoids useless routes altogether, by making straight for the hole. Frequent success has given this particular mode of behaviour an advantage, failure has suppressed the others : a clear, unequivocal and sufficiently definite connection between certain sense-impressions, and the successful mode of behaviour has now been established. One speaks of the ' pleasure of success ' and the ' *unpleasure* of failure,' but thereby oversteps the bounds even of the purely external (' objective ') method of approach, though, it is true, at a theoretically harmless point. If for the term ' feelings,' which we ourselves would experience in similar situations, is substituted anything else causally connected with success and failure, which can explain the opposite effects on memory, the difficulty is removed.

It is easily seen that for training (in its purest, primitive form) an ' overproduction of movements ', a ' trying-out ', is necessary so that there may be a certain amount of play for chance, which, as in throwing repeatedly at a goal or shooting with a shot-gun, is always to some extent concerned in exact successes. By forming a definite connection the amount of play which is left to chance is then gradually narrowed down and eventually excluded altogether. Thus a state is reached that might be compared to the instincts in respect of the fewness of the means employed and the sureness and precision of the achievement ; a state that can hardly be distinguished from a condition in which instincts alone are active, unless one knows its previous history. At this point we must approach the matter from an evolutionary point of view. (See §4 below.)

Trainableness is a property which has evolved to a fair degree of perfection only in the vertebrates. However, ants, bees and crayfish are susceptible to certain simple forms of training. How far fleas can really be trained, as it is said they can, I have never been able to determine satisfactorily. Fishes get accustomed to a particular feeding-place and gradually learn to avoid obstacles of a very simple kind, as in the case of the pike and the glass plate put in its pond. But that is not much. Nor do frogs and snakes belong to the animals readily able to learn. On the other hand many birds, such as falcons and parrots, can accomplish considerable feats and even the good old stupid hen can do a little. If out of a long row of grains of corn on a board every second grain is glued down, the hungry hen will at first go on pecking even at the ones she cannot pick up, but will gradually abandon these unsuccessful attempts and learn to take regularly only every second grain. The lesson is learnt so thoroughly that later on one need not glue down any of the grains, for the hen will only pick up every second one. The hen is even capable of this : one can glue every third grain ; after long training she learns to pick up always two and leave the third untouched.[1] Similarly it is said that if one takes some of the kittens from a cat's litter while the mother is away, leaving only one or two, on returning she immediately sets out to look for the missing ones, but if there are still three left, she does not miss any. That may be true : I do not know. Uncritical persons, who in psychological matters never hesitate to set up sweeping theories, would probably draw the conclusion that cats and hens can count up to three, but no further. No, such summary, simple explanations are no longer tolerated in animal psychology. As we shall see later in the case of the child, far more is necessary for real counting, for forming concepts of number, than the animals achieve here. Cats and hens can probably count neither up to three, nor up to two, nor —what is far more difficult—to one. But of this we shall have more to say later. Here we are concerned merely with the question of training. As I have mentioned, falcons, trained for hunting, and parrots, which can be taught to utter quite passably words and whole sentences, can accomplish more than hens. Mammals—we need only mention the horse, the elephant, the dog and the higher apes—go considerably further than birds. This course of development is unmistakably bound up with the rise of the cerebral cortex, or, put more accurately, with

---

[1] D. Katz and G. Révész, " Experimentellpsychologische Unter-suchungen mit Hühnern." *Z.Ps.* 50 (1909), 93.

the increased differentiation of certain quite definite regions of the cortex, known, on account of their probable function, as the association centres.

Man marches at the head of all the vertebrates. No other creature has to learn so much during life as he. Even if we leave out of account the multiplication table, the vocabularies of foreign languages and whatever else school and culture in general involve, this proposition holds good. Just think of what is necessary in order to learn the mother tongue, be this the most primitive of human languages known! And more still: man must acquire in the games of his earliest youth bodily dexterity, including grasping and all the most elementary manipulations. This training begins at once, in the first weeks of his life, when nature herself is his teacher. Later, adults who want to make the child one of them, take a hand; and finally the adolescent and the grown man, realizing the necessity for it and of their own free will, train themselves in all manner of ways. Every sports club has its ' trainers.' Every art, every trade, every science presupposes a certain fundamental knowledge which has to be mechanically acquired—and this, in principle, is simply training as we have defined it.

Another consideration: for animals capable of a higher degree of training, for those animals with ' plastic ' dispositions that can be moulded, nature has provided, in order to prepare them fully for the earnestness of life, a period of development in which they are more or less subject to the protection and example of their parents and of the other grown animals of their kind. This period is called youth; and most intimately connected with it are the games of youth. Young dogs and cats and the human child play, whereas beetles and insects, even the highly organised bees and ants, do not. This cannot be mere chance, but must rest upon an inner connection: *play supplements the plastic dispositions* and only together do they offer an equivalent for instincts. Play gives the long practice of which the unfinished, plastic dispositions are in need[1]; or, better still, it is itself this practice.

(c) *The Intellect.* Both teachers and pupils are well aware that all mechanical learning requires repetition, time, and practice, just as money is required for waging war. This, from the biological point of view, is the great disadvantage of training as opposed to instinct, which is ready for use from the beginning and functions with adequate perfection on the very first occasion. But what about a third function which combines the advantages of both instinct and training? Such a function has actually been provided for in the plan of evolution and is known as intellect. Robinson Crusoe on his island is a man whom the author constantly places in new situations. He does not run to and fro aimlessly like the hen before the garden fence until she chances on a hole; he does not go about trying things at random, but *makes discoveries by means of insight and reflection.* INVENTION, in the true sense of the term, is the biological achievement of intellect. Let us begin with the simplest case.

Suppose one confines a dog in a large, barred room and outside, a yard from the grating, one places a piece of meat, leaving inside the room a hooked stick or any other object by means of which the meat could be drawn in. What happens? Presumably the dog will not of himself think of employing the stick as a tool; he will whimper and howl, wander restlessly up and down in front of the grating, scratch at the bars, push his snout and paws out towards the meat, but will not reach the goal. If left to himself he would die of hunger within sight of food. Naturally it might be possible to train the dog to use the hooked stick, but that is not the same thing. The point at issue is whether and to what extent he can help himself. A man in the dog's position, even the most primitive, or a child of six, would have no

---

[1] Cf. Karl Groos, *Das Spiel*, Two essays; Jena, 1922. And Karl Bühler, *Die Krise der Psychologie*, 2nd Edition, Jena, 1928.

PLATE I

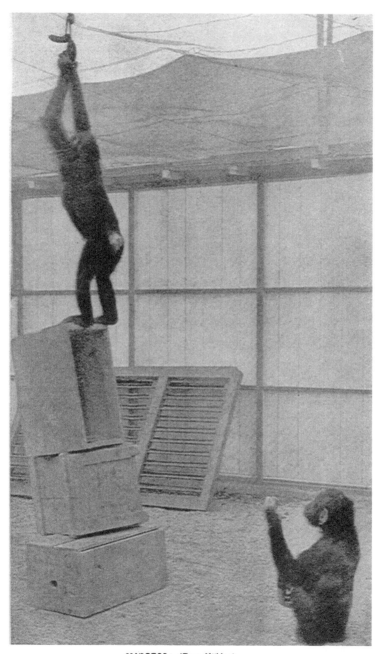

SUCCESS! (From Köhler.)

[face p. 10

difficulty here. MAN CREATES AND USES TOOLS ; ANIMALS DO NOT. That is a very old doctrine, founded on the most patent facts. But as we have recently learnt, it is not without exception, for the anthropoid apes also use tools and, in so far as the needs of the moment require them, create the most primitive tools themselves.

An investigation of W. Köhler, director of the German anthropoid station at Teneriffe, quite clearly proved this.[1] As everyone knows, the ape possesses, as the result of instinct and practice, marvellous dexterity in climbing, jumping and seizing. Now if a chimpanzee is put in a situation where fruit attracts him, but where the means he naturally has at his disposal do not suffice, he is still able to find a way out of the difficulty. Suppose the fruit is outside the grating of the experimental cage beyond reaching distance : what does he do ? From the branch of a tree, some plant-stalks, the top of a box, a piece of wire, he makes a stick to draw the fruit towards himself. If the fruit is hung high up, if there is no tree or wall to climb and no stick to be had, he drags a box along ; if necessary, he piles three, even four boxes one on top of the other, to grasp at the fruit from the top of his shaky tower or to bring it down with a leap (cf. Plate I). Some particularly remarkable achievements may be mentioned : fruit is placed outside the grating and a stick hung up in the cage. The chimpanzee with the aid of a box first gets the stick down and with this gets the fruit. Similarly, the animal is able to combine into a series two, three or even four separate actions with which it is already familiar, in order to achieve some definite purpose. Another case : a single bamboo stick is too short to reach the fruit outside, but there is another stick at hand, also short but thicker, open at both ends. In this situation the chimpanzees take both sticks, put them side by side so that often they partly cover each other, hold them carefully together with their hands and try to reach the fruit with the apparently

[1] Vide the references at the end of this Section.

lengthened stick, naturally without success. Sultan, the most gifted ape that Köhler studied, tormented himself in vain for hours in this attempt. At last he turned away from the grating, taking with him the two sticks. He sat down some distance away and began to play with them. Possibly by chance one went into the hole in the other and stuck there : the ape immediately realised his advantage, hastened back with the combined stick and got the fruit. Henceforth for him the problem of lengthening the sticks was solved and afterwards he would join even three sticks together. When there was nothing else at his disposal, he would split a lath with his sharp teeth and insert it into the hole. All this he did so clearly and decisively that the other animals, seeing what he did, were able to imitate him. (See Plate II.)

Köhler came to the conclusion that we can no longer refuse to admit that the apes have a kind of *primitive* ' insight,' but he was met by contradiction and doubt. It will depend on what we mean by ' insight.' The chimpanzee cannot as yet be in the position we are in when we think out some plan and clearly realise how one thing fits into another, or when we grasp the relation of end to means. He is as yet probably without concepts and the function of judgment. His thinking, in so far as there is something present which deserves that name, is restricted to short, unusually favourable moments of psychic high-tension. That is Köhler's opinion too. The rest of the argument would, in a lesser matter, scarcely demand further reflection ; but in this case far-reaching theoretical consequences would seem to be involved. I believe that certainty and insight in the exact sense of the term, are intimately connected with the function of judgment. I do not wish to do the apes an injustice ; but it seems to me that they have not as yet proved to us that they judge or can grasp connections in reasoning. The chimpanzee's discoveries look to me rather like happy *intuitions*. Let us remember that it is always merely a case of obtaining possession of an

PLATE II

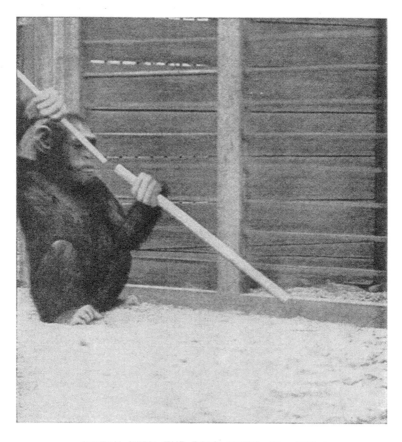

SULTAN WITH THE REED STICKS. (From Köhler.)

attractive fruit. It scarcely seems remarkable to us that the animal knows how to use branches for its ends, e.g., bending a branch to get at the fruit hanging on it, or breaking it off, striking with it, etc., as all this does not go beyond instinct and training. At any rate the correspondence between branch and fruit must be pretty well known to the tree-dweller. Now when he is sitting inside the experimental cage, with the branchless fruit outside and the fruitless branch inside, then from the psychological point of view, the main achievement is that he, as it were, brings them together perceptually or conceptually. The rest is self-evident. Similarly with the box : when the ape notices a fruit high up in the forest, nothing is more natural than that he should look about him for that tree trunk up which he has to climb to get at the fruit. In the cage there is a box in the field of vision instead of a tree and the psychic achievement consists in imagining this box placed at the proper spot. To wish and to do are then one, for the captive chimpanzee is always playing with boxes and dragging them about the place.

Whether this is so or not, the biological valuation of such achievements does not depend upon their detailed psychological explanation, nor on those questions which are as yet unanswered in this connection. In any case, there are these two facts to be considered : first, that in a new situation the chimpanzee will at first behave for several minutes or even hours exactly like the fowl at the garden fence, or the dog before the meat he cannot reach, until suddenly, very often only at the eleventh hour, when e.g., another ape outside comes suspiciously near the banana, a complete reaction takes place. The animal all at once grows calm and not infrequently sits still for a moment, its facial expression ' clears up ' and when it sets to work again after this the aimlessness and carelessness have been replaced by quiet, well-ordered behaviour, which in one attempt reaches the goal, often in a few seconds. Secondly, if the problem has been solved in this way only once, in future only a single attempt is necessary, i.e., the aimlessness of the first stage is not repeated. Such achievements do not, as opposed to everything we call training, require long and laborious practice.

These are two properties we can easily understand, because from our own experience we are well acquainted with them. One of the first scientific observations made in the psychology of thought processes on more difficult tasks was that very often the solution dawns upon us suddenly. Language has created a special interjection for this sudden ' inner illumination '—AHA ! Another, that has been clearly brought out in the examination of the thought processes of man and is perfectly well known from everyday life is : ONCE AND FOR ALL. A mathematical proof, for example, is not learnt by continued repetition, like a poem or a vocabulary. Or, to use a simpler example for the same distinction : the considerable difficulty and annoyance often caused by the manipulation of the lock of a trunk can either be got over by mere excited and aimless trying or by proceeding according to some plan and with partial insight. It is only in the second case that there is any likelihood of our getting on to the right track at once when the attempt is repeated.

If after a first satisfactory solution the external conditions are considerably altered, a third distinctive property becomes apparent in the achievements of the human intellect. I have in mind the following : The theorem of Pythagoras holds for all right-angled triangles, quite independently of their size, shape or position ; whoever has grasped the general meaning of the proverb " everyone is glad to give a falling wall a push " will at once recognize it again in quite a different dress, as in " even mice will bite dead cats " ; and when one has grasped the principle of the lever, one also understands the decimal balance. It would be extremely interesting to determine how far simple transferences, such as are necessary here, are present in the discoveries of the chimpanzee.

But enough of this. Even without this third property, the discoveries of the chimpanzee are sharply distinguished

from instinct and training by the other two. He is able
to do justice to new, unusual situations suddenly, perfectly
and as a rule once and for all, in a peculiar way; not by
trying, nor by acquiring rapidity and precision with
practice, but by an inner (psychic) process. This psychic
process is equivalent, as far as its results go, to those
processes which in ourselves we call *reflection*; quite
possibly in simpler cases it is no more than a kind of inner
groping, as it were, a (relatively) lively mechanism of
imaginal processes to which chance finds the key. Many
an invention and discovery of man takes place in the
same way.[1] And even if it has not as yet been conclusively
demonstrated whether beyond this the first traces of
methodical reflection and insight do occur in chimpanzees,
the biologist is justified in attributing to them ' intellect '
in his sense, since the ability to discover and invent is
precisely the specific achievement of this third stage in
mental development.

We cannot say to-day whether other of the higher
vertebrates, such as the dog, possess inventiveness,
so that there might be a possibility of tracing it by means
of more refined methods in still more primitive forms, or
whether invention plays an important part in the natural
life of the apes.   But there are facts which warn us against
over-estimating the achievements of the chimpanzees.
We know that no explorer has ever confused gorillas or
chimpanzees with men.   No traditional tools or methods
of using them differing from tribe to tribe (which would
point to the transmission from one generation to another
of some invention) have ever been found among them.
We do not know of any scratchings in sand or clay,
which would constitute a *representational drawing* or even
a mere ornament scribbled playfully, nor of any *representational language*, i.e., sounds signifying names. There
must be some inner reason for all this.

[1] Cf. O. Selz, *Die Gesetze der produktiven und unproduktiven Geistes-
tätigkeit*, Bonn, 1924; and O. Selz, " Die Gesetze der produktiven
Tätigkeit," *Arch. f. Psych.*, xvii (1913), 367 *et seq.*

(*d*). *History and appreciation of the theory of levels.*
Aristotle has anticipated us in the general idea of a
succession of levels in the psychic sphere. But only as
far as the general idea goes, for we proceed in a fundamen-
tally different fashion to-day. We leave the question as
to whether plants have souls completely out of account
and we do not set up a gulf between ourselves and the
animals. The object of our considerations is nothing
more than the patent usefulness of the activities of animal
and man. We accept the customary distinction between
the ready-made inheritance of the instincts, which are in
a high degree perfect but rigid, and the plastic adaptability
of the individual shown by the way in which animals can
be trained. To these we add the power of invention, a
third function deduced from our general knowledge of
human behaviour and the psychology of thought processes.
Our investigations of apes confirm these results. Thus
we have described our theme, but have by no means
exhausted the possibilities of research.

This research has three clearly recognizable ends in
view. First, to determine all the vast variety of forms in
which instinct, training, and intellect are realized and to
classify them neatly, as the botanist classifies his species.
Who would deny that there is *a whole world of types of
animal behaviour*, and that therefore everything called
instinct cannot be put into one bag ? The same holds for
training and learning. We know, for instance, that bees
and wasps can be ' accustomed ' to one feeding place, or,
to put it more accurately, they will return to some
profitable spot far from the nest and when they fly off,
circle round it in a way which suggests that they are
trying to memorize its position optically. But no one
will assume that one could train a bee, as one could a dog,
to approach a basin of sugar water only after it had
visited a near-by flower with no honey in it. The powers
of localization of the bee are most probably firmly built
into its instinctive functions, as it were predetermined by
their plan, and it has not yet been proved that associative

memory in the true sense of the term is involved. But at any rate from the lower animals up to the dog and even man there are manifold forms of learning. To these we have to add the biological varieties of intellect, about which science as yet knows almost nothing.

A second, and no less important, task is the investigation of the connection between the modes of behaviour and the bodily structure of animals. Compare the structural plan of the arthropoda with that of the vertebrates. On the one hand a skin like a coat of mail, an external, enveloping skeleton, which constitutes very unfavourable conditions for the development of flexibility ; on the other hand an axial skeleton offering unlimited possibilities for the development of joints. Does it not seem obvious that it is only the vertebrates which will profit by being provided with mental mobility ? There can be no doubt that an inner connection exists between these relations and that what is true for the broader differences will also hold for the finer ones.[1]

In the nervous system we see the highest expression of bodily structure and the direct *organ of the soul*. Among the insects a special part of the central nervous system, the ' fungiform body,' is strongly developed : the brain of the vertebrates contains an older as well as a more recent constituent, the palaencephalon and the neencephalon, and " examination of the animal kingdom has shown that the whole of the mechanism from the end of the spinal cord to the olfactory nerve, including the palaencephalon, is in principle similarly arranged in all higher and lower vertebrates, that is to say, the basis of the simplest functions is the same right through the series, in man as well as in the fishes " (Edinger). But the neencephalon superimposes itself on the palaencephalon as a new apparatus, beginning with the reptiles and growing rapidly, until in man it spreads like a large cloak over the whole of it. One will not go far wrong at first in regarding

[1] I heard this conception expounded in detail and with expert knowledge in a lecture by Professor Demoll in Munich.

this as going parallel with increasing trainability of the animal. There seem also to be anatomical facts in support of the assumption of a third level in the structure of the human brain. In the anthropoid apes, and far more so in man, one finds a new increase in the relative weight of the brain, which takes place chiefly in the cortex. New fields with rich fibre connections in all directions are developed in the cortex and pushed in between the old ones, in man above all the infinitely important centres for speech.

Natura non facit saltum, development proceeds continuously, is a well-founded doctrine. To assume that our idea of a structural series of levels or stages is opposed to it, would be to misunderstand us. It seems to me that in our third task, the psychological estimation of animal behaviour, we have to proceed far more carefully than is often the wont to-day. Since E. Hering expressed it as his carefully considered opinion that memory, in the widest sense of the term, is a fundamental property of all organic matter, the doctrine of the *mneme* has been elaborated with many a fine name borrowed from the Greek. It may be that instinct and training rest on this same common basic principle ; it may be, in fact it is even probable, that in the original natural state of affairs there is a certain amount of free play as regards the indefiniteness of reactions and the capacity of the individual to get into firmer grooves, and that the partly real, partly merely apparent rigidity of the complicated instincts is a secondary characteristic. Even if one has a certain justification for speaking of ' race-memory,' ' race-training,' and calling instincts ' inherited habits '—although many a problematic assumption is involved in this, such as that acquired characteristics can be transmitted—one does not thereby remove the obvious differences between instinct and training. At least the line of development is different in each and in the vast field of biological existence it will be as in the small history of the mind of man, where we can trace historically that to a new direction in development there corresponds a new ' mentality.' Greater still, and fraught with graver consequences, was the innovation of inventiveness. And again we can see no break with the past. This new great step forward was perhaps introduced merely by a small advance in conceptualization or a somewhat freer play of associations. The point is *that proper use had to be made of it.* In the biological range we know of no intermediate links between the mentality of the chimpanzee and that of man, but we can trace the development of the human child. There we shall see how the transition takes place.

REFERENCES

C. L. MORGAN, *Instinct and Experience* (1910) ; L. EDINGER, *Einführung in die Lehre vom Bau und den Verrichtungen des Nervensystems* (2nd edn., 1912) ; W. KÖHLER, *The Mentality of Apes*, (2nd edn., 1925) ; CH. BÜHLER, " Das Problem des Instinktes," *Zeitschr. f. Psychol.*, CIII (1927).

2.—ON THE INHERITANCE OF INTELLECTUAL QUALITIES.

(a) *The Mendelian Laws.* The experiments which the Augustine monk (later abbot) Gregor Mendel, carried out on the hybridization of plants have been the egg of Columbus for the doctrine of heredity. By the definiteness of his experimental method Mendel compelled nature to give an unequivocal answer to his question. What will happen if I cross only once, two individual plants of closely related species, differing merely in a certain easily recognizable property like the colour of the flower, and then allow the progeny to multiply by self-fertilization ? Mendel decided this experimentally. The simple, quantitative formulation and theoretical interpretation of his results constitute the famous *Mendelian laws of heredity.* Their quantitative expression is so simple in uncomplicated cases, that it can be explained to any schoolchild. It is like the multiplication table. If I multiply two odd numbers, the product is also an odd number ; if I multiply two even numbers, or an odd number with an even one, the product is even. But suppose the product is formed in not quite so obvious a way, from the factors (a, b) x (a, b) after one of the elements, either a or b, has been cancelled. If chance is the factor deciding which shall be cancelled, then there are four probabilities for the product : a x a ; a x b ; b x a ; b x b. If a is the odd, b the even element, then in $\frac{1}{4}$ of the cases the product will be odd, in $\frac{3}{4}$ even. We have exactly the same in the multiplication table from 1 to 100 : $\frac{1}{4}$ of the products is odd, $\frac{3}{4}$ are even. The other cases need hardly be discussed: (a, a) x (b, b) and (a, b) x (b, b) will only give even products, (a, a) x (a, b) will give half even and half odd.

These are precisely the numerical relations which Mendel found ; the problem was to explain them. Odd, even, and multiplication have, of course, nothing to do with the process of heredity ; they are merely illustrative analogies to make the matter clear in a few words. In sexual propagation a new individual arises out of the union of the egg-cell of the mother and the sperm-cell of the father. In the nuclear substance of both cells, the material carrier of the inheritance, well-known and delicately differentiated processes take place, which, before their union, correspond to the cancelling in the above numerical analogy and afterwards to the formation of products. *The child receives exactly one half of its inheritance from its father, exactly the other half from its mother and it is so arranged that father and mother participate equally in laying the basis for every single quality inherited by the child.* Now the obvious fact, which seems to contradict this proposition, that in certain things the child ' takes after ' its father more and in others more after its mother, rests upon very important facts, the understanding of which is of supreme importance. First there are the facts of *suppression* of hereditary characters. One cannot tell offhand, without calculation, whether an even number chosen at random is the product of two even numbers, or of one odd and one even number. Now when Mendel crossed red-flowering with white-flowering peas, he got only red-flowering " children " in the first generation. That the white-flowering character of one parent had not been lost, but was suppressed or " latent," was clearly shown in the succeeding generations. The qualities of the red flower are in this case *dominant*, those of the white *recessive*. A suppressed hereditary character always manifests itself in the further course of heredity when the dominating influence which suppressed it is *split off*. This is the second fundamental fact. It is not true to say that each individual carries with it all the characters of

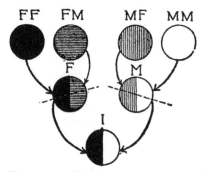

FIG. 1.—DIAGRAM OF HEREDITY ACCORDING TO MENDEL.

its ancestors. Fig. 1 shows us the true state of affairs. An individual (I) inherits exactly half from its father (F) and the other half from its mother (M). These on their part only transmit half of what they themselves received from their parents, so that there is no cumulative effect. The other half has been 'split off' from its gonads before these united to form a new individual. In our diagram the whole of the hereditary influences which might have been exerted on I from the father's mother (FM) and the mother's father (MF) have been cancelled out. In practice this extreme case will rarely be found. The splitting off in F and M, as indicated by the dotted lines, will take place in countless different ways. But it will at once come to mind that one child may be " exactly like his grandfather on the father's side " or like any other of the four grandparents, or it may have none of the characteristics of one or other of them. In this way exceptional intellectual qualities in a family may be lost, or physical and mental defects and abnormities be eliminated completely.

It will be readily seen that wherever such simple relations of dominance exist, every individual in whom a recessive character appears at all, must be regarded as being pure-bred with respect to this character—just as one can say immediately of any odd number that it can have no even number as factor. Thus in man brown eyes dominate blue ; two blue-eyed parents can therefore never have children with brown eyes, whereas brown-eyed parents, in whom the other disposition is latent, can very well have blue-eyed children. But we must not imagine that this simple law of dominance holds good for all characteristics ; on the contrary, the progress of research has shown that extremely complicated relations exist and it would seem that Mendel was extraordinarily fortunate in his choice of experimental subjects. If elsewhere in nature two differently directed ' influences ' are brought together, the result is generally a mixture and the same holds true for the hereditary process : red and white, for instance, resulting in pink. Moreover, any single manifest characteristic is often dependent on another or on many others, so that it cannot be changed at will. Finally, in special cases there are many other circumstances as well which complicate matters. One of the factors in our calculations is ' chance,' which merely means that we do not know *all* the effective factors.

(*b*). *Investigations on Man.* The Mendelian laws have been proved to hold for a very large number of physical and a few mental characters. We can circumvent the difficulty that experiments on heredity in man cannot be carried out, by utilizing the cases which nature herself offers us and tabulating similar qualities. But it is more difficult in the case of mental traits, to obtain reliable data over three generations in any particular case. There are two methods of approach, each of which has its advantages and disadvantages : we can either utilize determinations which have already been made for other purposes, or we can have new ones made *ad hoc*. Should the latter plan ever be properly carried out, it would need a great deal of preliminary psychological investigation, much scientific tact and a ready grasp of what can be determined with certainty and what can be regarded as more or less constant, fundamental characteristics, not to speak of a large staff of trained observers. I imagine that in more settled times, the necessary voluntary workers will be found among our clergymen, teachers and doctors.

Meanwhile let me say a few words about what has been achieved by the first method. In general, not much is recorded about the mental traits of the average civilized human being. We shall hardly get anything out of the registers of births and marriages. But in the case of certain characteristics deviating from the norm, the lunatic asylums offer interesting material, which, with a little care and ingenuity, can be supplemented so that in a sufficiently large number of families the hereditary course of the mental disease can be traced through three or even more generations. It is only fairly recently that psychiatry has exchanged old, deeply rooted conceptions for the fundamental modern doctrines of heredity, but the progress of research seems to be more rapid now. It has been shown to be probable that in the case of a certain group of mental diseases to which *dementia praecox* belongs, there are specific hereditary dispositions that " mendelize" in a relatively simple way and are recessive with respect to the normal dispositions. We see rather more clearly in the case of another complex of tendencies which lead, not to the asylum, but to prison. There are people who from youth have an ineradicable inclination towards thieving and vagabondage and who in later life become constant guests of prisons and convict stations. They possess a fatal heritage, which is handed on from generation to generation in obedience to the same laws that regulate the transmission of any bodily characteristic and which is recessive with respect to normal tendencies. It must be remembered, however, that only in the case of men does this tendency give rise to actions ending in gaol with the frequency required by the Mendelian laws. Examining the genealogies of about a hundred such individuals we have found :

TABLE I

PARENTS	SONS OF CONVICTABLE AGE		
	n.	of these convicted.	
		Found	Calculated.
Both convicted - -	30	28=93.5%	100%
One convicted, the other tainted - - -	177	89=50.3%	50%

As convictions in our sense only hard labour or long term sentences were taken into account ; the two individuals of the first group who had escaped severe penalties up to the time of this investigation were also vagabonds in character, but somewhat more harmless and cautious than the others.

Of particular interest for the doctrine of mental development is the question as to the inheritance of intellectual gifts. Here we have a work of W. Peters[1] along Mendelian lines, who used material from the schoolroom. From the extant annual school reports Peters has compared the marks gained by children, parents and grandparents, an undertaking which can be carried through only in council schools of villages with a relatively permanent population. Now school marks are certainly no pure criterion of intelligence, for apart from the human weaknesses and imperfect judgment of the teacher, they depend on various

[1] W. PETERS, " über Vererbung psychischer Fähigkeiten," *Fortschritte der Psychol. u. ihre Anwendung*, III, 1915.

external, helpful or disturbing environmental factors and the assiduity of the child, or, in general, on its adaptation to school conditions and its " will to learn." Nevertheless, Peters, using a statistical method, with the help of ideal critical circumspection and auxiliary investigations of his own, was able to eliminate all secondary factors so completely that we may accept his results as being well established. Chief among them is the law of alternating inheritance of degrees of intelligence, that is, if one of the parents is exceptionally clever and the other more than normally dull, the children as a rule do not form an average, but take after either the one or the other parent. Which of them, it is not possible to say off-hand, because of the obscure, complicated conditions of human breeding. But even when a relatively pure-bred dullard mates with a relatively pure-bred bright wit, it seems that now the one and then the other influence is the stronger. We are in all probability not dealing here with simple characteristics at all

In a word, some of the simple physical characteristics which have been investigated in plants, animals, and man, are transmitted quite independently of one another. If one assumed such an independence for all dispositions, the whole heritage of an individual could be considered purely as a mosaic, out of which every stone can be taken and replaced by a corresponding one of another colour. This deduction should raise objections. For in the finished individual we recognize everywhere connections, correlations between various characteristics. The visible characteristics of the individual can therefore hardly form a merely additive whole, but must give rise to more or less well-ordered systems, unities of higher and lower degrees. And it is unlikely that the hidden hereditary dispositions form a mosaic. In the exact sense of that term this assumption does not seem to be probable, although it is not quite as undebatable as may appear to some of us at first sight. For we see that much of the uniformity in the bodily and mental development through which we pass had first to be acquired, while we carry many a conflict about with us which is never overcome. If, therefore, it appears that the unitary aspects of the highest complex qualities of the individual are not present once and for all from the beginning, but are capable of development, then it seems probable that the lower ones also have to establish themselves in the struggle of conflicting tendencies. They, too, are not given once and for all from the beginning. At any rate Mendel's thesis that the hereditary dispositions are independently replaceable has this in its favour, that it has been shown to hold good for a large number of attributes.

(c). *Practical application.* Sugar-beet, corn, apples, dogs, horses, goats, are bred with the greatest success according to the laws of the modern doctrine of heredity and it is only for his own species that man has yet failed to take advantage of them. While appreciating quite soberly the practical resistances in the way, one can yet wish fervently that some of them may gradually be removed. If only a little could be done to reduce the population of homes for incurables—bodily and mental— lunatic asylums and prisons, the efforts of 'eugenics' would be fully justified. Personally I believe that what is needed at the present time more than violent changes in legislation is the advancement of science and the dissemination of its results among teachers, ministers, doctors and social workers.

REFERENCES

W. JOHANNSEN, *Elemente der exakten Erblichkeitslehre*, 2nd edn., 1914. C. CORRENS, *Die neuen Vererbungsgesetze*, 1912. L. PLATE, *Vererbungslehre, mit besonderer Berücksichtigung des Menschen, für Studierende, Ärzte und Züchter*, 1913. BAUER, LENZ, FISCHER, *Menschliche Erblichkeitslehre*, 2nd edn., Munich, 1922, 2 vols. C. RATH, "Uber die Vererbung von Dispositionen zum Verbrechen," *Münchener Studien zur Philos. und Psychol.*, Heft 2, 1914. W. PETERS, "Uber Vererbung psychischer Fähigkeiten," *Fortschritte d. Psychol.* III. (1915) (with full references to the Bibliography). *idem*, "Vererbung und Persönlichkeit" (*Sammel referat*), *VIII. Kongress f. exp. Psych.*, Jena 1924. *idem*, *Die Vererbung geistiger Eigenschaften und die psychische Konstitution*, Jena, 1925. R. GOLDSCHMIDT, *Einführung in die Vererbungswissenschaft*, 3rd edn., Leipzig, 1920.

3.—AIMS AND METHODS OF CHILD-PSYCHOLOGY.

(*a*). *History.* The modern study of the child is of German origin. From about the middle of the 19th century, German doctors and teachers started a movement which, on the somatic side, was first put on a sound basis and unified into a system by K. Vierordt in his " *Physiologie des Kindesalters,*" (1881) and on the psychological side by W. Preyer in his " *Seele des Kindes,*" (1882). Preyer's book has become the fundamental work in child-psychology and the source of an extraordinarily assiduous activity in this field, in which all the civilized nations, particularly the United States, have participated.

It is a remarkable book, full of interesting and conscientious observations, but poor in original ideas. In philosophical quarters one could hear that unpleasant phrase " nursery-psychology." It was, perhaps, not quite unfounded ; but employed without qualification, it was a shining example of that kind of short-sightedness particularly ill-becoming to the philosopher. True, the undertaking was a bold one : to go to the nursery with the problems of humanity and attempt to advance our knowledge of them with no other aids than those of exact observation and meticulous registration of the thousand apparently long-known trivialities of child-life. That sort of thing is well calculated to disconcert many of those who are not able to see beyond the narrow confines of properly circumscribed and traditional methods in some specialized subject. But it ought not to upset the philosopher, whose profession it is to know the value of method and its rise from primitive beginnings.

Anyhow, Preyer, carried along by the vigorous spirit of ' physiological ' psychology, has managed to prevail. He himself was no pioneer in psychology ; he has given us neither new methods nor a new law of psychic activity ; but he rendered lasting service in grasping the new field as a whole at the most favourable moment and tilling it with scientific care down to the smallest detail. Even to-day his book is a mine of observations, which one seldom searches in vain for facts bearing on any question. But when it comes to theoretical interpretation, general points of view and ideas, we can and must make more rigorous demands to which the popular psychology of Preyer is no longer equal. Others have arisen who have surpassed and replaced it. I need mention in each case only the most important : On the first steps in mental development, Baldwin, Miss Shinn, Major, Dearborn, and W. Dix ; on language, Ament, Meumann and Stern ; on play, imagination and thinking, Groos and others ; on drawing, which in Preyer's scheme had as yet no place, there exists a very big literature.

(b). *Aims.* The science of the child, too, claims the proud privilege of every pure science—to investigate its objects for its own sake. True, the child is more to us than stones, plants and animals. It is of us, the heir to our culture, a growing personality over which we watch with the care of physician or priest and which we regard with the eyes of responsible teachers. In it, the history of our thought is recapitulated and continued, so that we can try to understand ourselves better and take cognizance of future currents of thought. The student of prehistory will turn to it too, when he has realized that no one can offer him more towards replacing the lost first records of humanity's progress to civilization, than his own child can when it is properly understood. If we simply bring them together like this, we get a somewhat mixed company of problems and interests. So we shall carefully select some of the already recognizable aspects of applied child-psychology, but each specialist will have to study the most important for himself. Our chief concern will be the understanding of the great phases and laws of development. We shall direct our attention in the first place to the *structural laws* manifesting themselves during the course of development and secondly to the *causes*, the dynamic forces, which modify it in this way or that. When a gardener sows mixed seeds in a flower bed, each will sprout and grow for itself, regardless of the others ; and only the struggle for food, light and air will bring about an equilibrium. In the organism, however, there is no such anarchy, but strictly regulated interdependence : memory is dependent on attention, the will on affects and judgments etc. So it will not be sufficient to follow the development of every single basic function of the mind by itself. We must also come to realize their mutual dependence, their so-called 'correlations.' There can be no doubt to-day that there is a perfectly stable inner rhythm of mental growth, which can be helped or hindered by external influences, but never quite destroyed. To achieve an understanding of it, will be to have the deepest insight into the mental structure of man which is allowed us and of which we are capable. That in itself is a tremendous task.

The second field of endeavour, the determination of causes, is no smaller. Inflammations of the pia mater and diseases of the thyroid gland can cause idiocy ; on the other hand cured hydrocephaly may sometimes leave behind conditions favourable to the growth of the brain. But if we wish to trace out the framework of the normal process, we must, for the time being, leave out of account such influences of disease and bodily defects, however interesting and instructive they may be in themselves. We have spoken of heredity ; the child, whom we are investigating, brings with him bodily constitution and hereditary dispositions, and a part of the wide individual differences are to be put down to their account. Nor is the sex of the child a matter of indifference. The other differences between child and child are derived from the influences acting upon them from the outside. There we have the unintentional effects of the *milieu* into which the individual is born, the physical and psychic *milieu*, with its social, national, and religious atmosphere. Finally there are the intentional influences of education. Special insight and training are necessary for disentangling the common characteristics of 'the child' from the rich confusion of individual detail, but as the general problems

appear more and more clearly, so this will become easier
Then will be the time to reintroduce systematically into
the sphere of investigations, those factors that we neglected
at the beginning.

(c). *Methods.* We should be taking a prejudiced view
if we believed that really exact results in the mental
sphere can be obtained only by experiment. The older
school of biology, (I need only mention Darwin), discovered
notable facts even without experiment. Child-psychology
has been, and is to some extent still, in a similar position,
Preyer introduced the *diary method* and found many
imitators. At first everything about the child seemed
new, interesting and worth noting down : the pen could
hardly keep up with the observations. The early observers
would have liked to preserve the entire drama without a
gap, by means of film and phonograph, which, luckily,
were not in existence at that time. Luckily, that is, for
the children under observation, for even to-day science
can derive much benefit from child biographies, as detailed
as possible, provided the individual circumstances are
recorded with the necessary psychological circumspection
and accuracy. How that is to be done, it is not easy to say
in two words, or with equal correctness for all cases. He
who earnestly desires to gain a deeper understanding of
the greatest of all the dramas of evolution, the growing to
human estate of our children, must be prepared to realize
that this is impossible without very thorough preparations.
As in every science and art, one has first to learn to see, in
order to be able to understand more than a good nurse does.
The times in which the concepts of popular psychology
sufficed are past. How meagre appears to us at the
present time what even the greatest of the pioneers of
pedagogy, Comenius, Rousseau, Pestalozzi, had to say
about the first years of the child ! Fröbel, I think, is in
many respects an exception.

The systematic introduction of the child to artificial
situations in the first years of its life is effected chiefly in
the form of animal, or, as we might style it more generally,

of *achievement-experiments :* The observer tries to determine what a living organism is able to accomplish, to *achieve,* under given conditions, whether it be bodily or mental acts that are involved. The direct information which such an experiment gives, is merely whether a problem can be solved and what the limits of capacity in this particular case, are, *vide* the experiments of Köhler with chimpanzees. When the animal is hungry and sees fruit, the food seeking instinct is called into action : it has to be determined whether and how the animal is able, by a mental act, to overcome obstacles that are introduced. We have to proceed similarly in the case of the child, i.e. we must create those simplified and transparent conditions under which it first gives itself up completely to the achievement of the end and which secondly, permit us to tell with certainty when the reaction has failed and to give the psychological reason for this. The real driving force of the mental process will in most cases be presupposed and not examined more closely, as in our example of hunger and the food seeking instinct. Elsewhere acquired habits and the will of the child are called into play as, when I say to a two-year-old, " *fetch* this," " *do* that." In all cases the experimenter's first care must be to give the necessary impetus to the instinctive forces and guide them in the same direction, so that failure, or a mistake may not be wrongly attributed to a lack of ability. Very many otherwise well conceived experiments on children and animals have foundered on this rock. It stands to reason that the aim of the investigation may also be the releasing of some psychic mechanism—starting up the motor, as it were—or involve one of the directional factors. I include in this, investigations such as that of the reflexes of the newborn child and should like to suggest the term *release experiments* for them. Thus Kussmaul[1] has determined the reactions of the newborn babe to sweet, sour and bitter liquids, which are placed on

[1] *Untersuchungen über das Seelenleben des Neugeborenen Menschen,* 1859.

its tongue (cf. p. 428). Sweet liquids start a sucking and swallowing action, whereas bitter or sour ones lead to opening of the mouth and active ejection, in which the whole of the muscles round the mouth take part every time and give the face its characteristic ' expression ' for sweetness, sourness or bitterness. The old designation of *expression-experiment* is appropriate when we are concerned with mimicry and other concomitant phenomena of psychic states as well as the connections between the two. It obviously lies in the nature of the case that there must be gradual transitions between these two types of experiment.[1]

But there is one thing which all these methods have in common : the psychic factors, which in the last resort are the things that matter, have to be deduced from other results that the experiment gives us. It cannot be otherwise even in child-psychology, for the little ones are not able to make more delicate *introspections ;* their activities are as yet chiefly directed towards the outside world. A categorical denial would, however, be premature ; the French investigator Binet, has proved by means of many excellent experiments, that with patience and critical care valuable statements about conceptual processes and acts of thought can be drawn even from children of less than compulsory school age.

We have not yet exhausted the methods. The whole of Wundt's *Völkerpsychologie* is based on psychological *interpretation*, i.e., the interpretation and explanation of the so-called ' objective mental structures,' language, art, customs and laws, which the human mind has created for itself. In the chapters on the language and drawings of children we shall follow similar paths and the recent investigations of fairy tales will show us a not unimportant variation of the same method.

(d). *The limits of child-psychology, and the phases of childhood.* We cannot extend the programme indefinitely.

---

[1] Cf. Bühler, *Die Krise der Psychologie*, for a discussion as to the justification and compatibility of various psychological methods.

From a biological point of view childhood is at an end on the completion of puberty. Moreover, the aim of our investigations is not the individual as such, but general laws. Biography, the history of single personalities, is a different matter. I am in complete agreement with Dilthey, Windelband, Rickert and others in so far as they emphasize the individual value of the history of personality. But I think, as matters stand to-day, that it would be presumptuous for the scientist who tries to discover general laws, to attempt to usurp the functions of the historian. For we cannot now (and in all probability shall never be able to) conceive of personality as the calculable product of those influences which have helped to build it up. Nevertheless we, too, must demand understanding and respect for our type of search after casual laws. *The process of mental development is also subject to laws.* It is always most annoying in the war of methods and principles, when the other side tries to set up what it imagines to be *a priori*, immovable boundaries. We have already achieved something and will, no doubt, achieve more.

The biggest steps in the development of the human mind are taken in the first years and it is on these, therefore, that the chief interest of our science will be largely concentrated, just as it is mainly embryos that are examined in connection with the doctrines about the development of the body. Pedagogy will do well to drive its psychological pillar down as far as this ; it will not fare worse than the medical art, which devotes a large part of its disciples' time to the first phases in the development of the body, because it has realized that the fundamental laws of development must be learnt from the simplest circumstances, where they appear most clearly. The nursery, lunatic asylums, and schools for the mentally deficient, are places where one can learn most about the structure of the human mind and the general lines of its development. It is only the years of adolescence, in which the child grows into the man or woman, which can to some extent be compared with the importance and the force of events in the first years of life.

The division of the period of development will ultimately have to follow the same principle which intuitively led some pedagogue of the past to coin the phrases, *first or silly quarter, the grabber, the toddler, the babbler.* That is to say, the phases will be determined by what happens to be in the forefront of developmental progress. For it is often the case that the energy of mental growth concentrates itself on some single point, on some definite group of similiar activities. We shall not infrequently emphasize and name such phases, e.g., the chimpanzee age of the infant, the stage of asking names, asking why, the Struwwelpeter-age, fairy-tale-age, Robinson-Crusoe-age, etc. The first fundamental attempt at rigorous systematization is made in the book by Charlotte Bühler : *Kindheit und Jugend, Grundgesetze der seelischen Entwicklung.* Leipzig, 1928.

REFERENCES

(1) As general expositions of the psychology of the child, the following works can be recommended :—W. PREYER, *Die Seele des Kindes,* 1882, 7th edn., 1908, 424 pp.   J. SULLY, *Studies of Childhood,* 1895, new edn., 1903.   K. GROOS, *Das Seelenleben des Kindes,* 6th edn., 1923, 312 pp.   W. STERN, *The Psychology of Early Childhood,* 4th edn., 1928. K. BÜHLER, *Die geistige Entwicklung des Kindes,* 5th edn., 1929. CH. BÜHLER, *Kindheit u. Jugend. Genese des Bewusstseins,* Leipzig, 1928, 307 pp.   KOFFKA, K., *The growth of the Mind.*
(2) Historical :   W. AMENT, " Eine erste Blütezeit der Kinderpsychologie um die Wende des 18 zum 19. Jahrhundert," *Zeitsch. f. pädag. Psychol.* IX. (1907), idem, *Fortschritte der Kinderseelenkunde.* 1895-1903, 2nd edn. 1906 (contains abstracts and a valuable survey of the literature). H. GÖTZ, " Zur Geschichte der Kinderpsychologie und der experimentellen Pädagogik, *Zeitsch. f. pädag. Psychol.* XIX, 1918.   CH. BÜHLER and H. HETZER, *Zur Problemgeschichte der Kinderpsychologie.*
(3) Methods :   C. STUMPF, " zur Methodik der Kinderpsychologie," *Zeitsch. f. pädag. Psychol.,* II. (1900).   STANLEY HALL, *Aspects of Child Life and Education,* New York, 1921.   D. KATZ, " Studien zur Kinderpsychologie," *Wissenschaftl. Beiträge z. Pädagogik u. Psychol.,* 4 *Heft,* 1913.
(4) Effects of environment :   Of recent works I need only mention ARGELANDER, A., " Der Einfluss der Umwelt auf die geistige Entwicklung," *Jenaer Beitr. z. Erziehungs u. Jugendpsy.,* 7, 1928.   BUSEMANN, A., *Pädagogische Milieukunde,* Halle, 1927.   HETZER, H., *Kindheit und Armut, psychol. Methoden der Armutsforschung und Armutsbekämpfung,* Leipzig, 1929. All three works contain many references to the literature.

4.—THE PHYSICAL DEVELOPMENT OF THE CHILD

In the nine months of embryonic development, the body of the child grows from the fertilized ovum, a body microscopically minute. It is born in human form with a weight of three to four kilograms. All the important

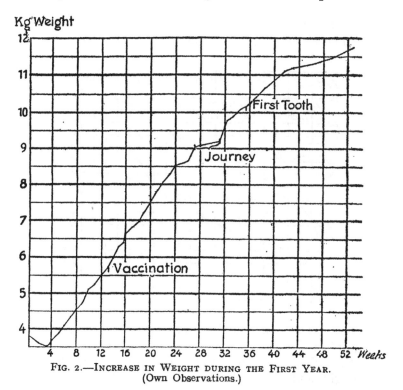

FIG. 2.—INCREASE IN WEIGHT DURING THE FIRST YEAR.
(Own Observations.)

organs are present in the newborn child, the organic systems are ready in outline and there almost seems to be only one thing left for this little being to do—*to grow*. Almost, for certain inner transformations have still to be carried out : the skeleton is largely cartilaginous and has to ossify before it can fully perform its functions ; the teeth are missing ; some organs which have already reached the summit of their development, disappear altogether, like the thymus gland, or, like the marrow of the bones, which originally serves to form red blood corpuscles, lose their specific function. But far more important for our purposes than all this, is the development of the brain, that organ on which the mental processes are directly dependent. Even after birth great transformations take place in it.

Let us consider, briefly, these matters in turn.

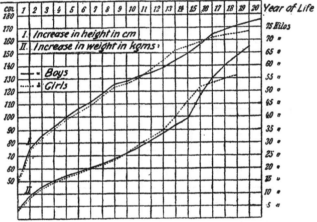

FIG. 3.—THE GROWTH OF THE BODY. (After *Biedert-Selter*.)

(*a*). *The total growth of the body*. Fig. 2 represents graphically the increase in weight of a girl in the first year of her life. This child was born with a relatively high weight and, although she was fed on the bottle, was fortunate enough to escape any serious illness. It is plain how regularly the body grows when external disturbances are absent. Fig. 3 represents average values obtained from selected healthy and strong children of German and Dutch families of the higher classes ; they are somewhat higher than those found for children of other races and the poorer classes of the population. But the laws of growth are the same everywhere : after the rapid rise of the curves in the first years, we notice a second period of growth in the second decade, which sets in at the age of puberty and consequently somewhat earlier in girls than in boys. In their eleventh year girls are ahead of boys of the same age and they obtain a considerable start in the next few years, to fall permanently behind later. Finer details are naturally lost in average curves, so we find that a third period of accelerated growth,

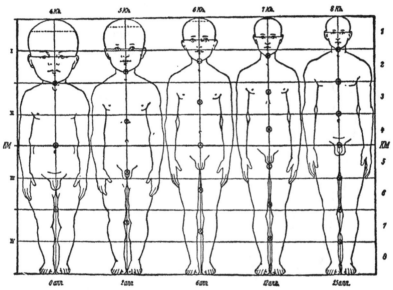

FIG. 4.—THE DEVELOPMENT OF THE BODILY PROPORTIONS. (After *Stratz*.)

which as a rule falls between the eighth and ninth years, is hardly indicated in these. The entry into school generally brings with it a transitory set-back, which occasionally is fatal to weak and sickly children, but is compensated for in healthy children by an energetic reaction. Careful individual curves, obtained from frequent measurements, show a '*natural rhythm of growth*,' in which a 'stretching' of the body precedes the biggest increase in weight. This was also found in cases where the body makes up lost ground after lengthy periods of

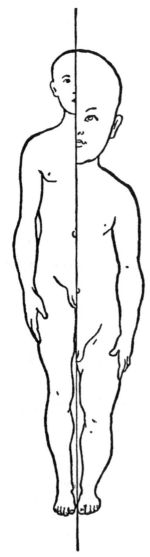

FIG. 5.—THE BODILY PROPOR-
TIONS OF THE NEW-BORN
INFANT AND THE ADULT.
(After *Stratz*.)

arrested development. Even in animal curves, based on daily measurements, this rhythm was apparent : the main period falls into spring and early Summer, whilst the main increase in weight takes place in late Summer and autumn, after which a phase of general minimal growth closes the annual cycle in the later winter months. (Malling-Hansen).

(b). *Changes in the bodily proportions.* The most important readjustments of relative bodily proportions can be seen from Figs 4 and 5. The relation of the length of the trunk to the length of the arms remains nearly constant, as does the relation of these two lengths to the total length of the body. On the other hand the relative height of the head and length of the legs increases. Fig. 4 shows the proportions of the new-born, 2-, 6-, 12-year old child and of the 25 year old man, where the total height of the body is respectively 4, 5, 6, 7 and 8 times the height of the head. It must be remembered, however, that the classic proportions of the Greeks allowed the height of the body of a grown man to be only $7\frac{2}{3}$ times that of the head. In the adult, the length of the legs is about half that of the total length, in a new-born infant scarcely one third. The cranium is chiefly responsible for the relatively enormous size of the head of a new-born child, while the facial parts are as yet quite insignificant ; the two toothless jaws are diminutive. A horizontal line drawn through the pupils of the eyes just halves the height of the head in an adult ; in the new-born child it divides it in the ratio 5 : 3.

Finally we note the changes in the measurements of the chest, which in infants appears relatively more vaulted in front, narrowed across and opened like a funnel towards the bottom, and the changes due to upright carriage : a normal curvature of the originally straight spine, inclination and broadening of the pelvis and a slight depression of the diaphragm and internal organs. We remind the reader, too, of the development of secondary sexual characters, which takes place during puberty : the sprouting of the beard in the male and of the pubic hair in both sexes ; the changes in the thorax, which determine the ' breaking ' of the voice ; the development of the breasts, broadening of the pelvis and general rounding off of the bodily contours in the female. We have now enumerated all the important adjustments in the bodily proportions.

(c). *The development of the brain.* The facts with regard to the perfecting of the most important and the only immediate organ of the soul are as follows : of the two parts of the central nervous system, one, the spinal cord, is structurally almost complete at birth, functions in nearly all of its parts and merely needs to grow. Only the so-called pyramidal paths, which serve to conduct motor impulses from the brain, are not quite ready to function. The second part on the other hand, the brain, although possessing considerable size and its specific shape, is only ready for functioning in those parts which are functionally related to the spinal cord. To these belong, for example, the centres for the automatic regulation of breathing and the circulation of the blood, without which the child would be incapable of living, as well as a number of other centres for vital processes. They all lie in the brain stem below the cortex and are therefore called subcortical centres.

The cortex itself has the external appearance it has in the adult, i.e. it has all its convolutions and sulci and even all the ganglion or nerve cells. An increase in the number of nerve cells does not take place anywhere after birth. What is lacking, is their ramified continuations which, in their totality, constitute the conducting paths of nervous processes. In some parts of the brain these nerve-continuations have not yet grown out of the cells at all, in others they are provided, but lack the isolating sheaths of perineurium, which later surround every single fibre, and are therefore not yet ready to function. The development of the medullary sheaths is called the ' *maturing process of the nerve fibres* ' and it has been possible to trace the time of maturing of the various systems of fibres in minute detail. At birth, only those paths are provided with sheaths, which lead from the sense organs to the cortex (sensory paths) ; they have developed in the last embryonal months, first for the sense of touch and the muscle sense, almost simultaneously for the senses of smell and taste, later for the sense of sight and last for the sense of hearing. The large motor paths, on the other hand, which arise at the cortex and later conduct the will impulses to the muscles, show merely the first signs of maturity, whilst in the manifold connecting paths of the cerebral centres below these, not even this is visible.

There can be no doubt that accurate knowledge of these developmental processes in the brain is of prime importance for understanding the enormous mental progress of the child in its first years. Indeed, interesting facts have been discovered about the brains of completely idiotic children : development had been arrested on very primitive levels ; in some cases only very few nerve processes had been developed, in others those that had been developed had again been destroyed and in a third group there had been no development of conducting paths. We may hope that it will be possible to find, in the structural development of the cerebral cortex, similar causes for certain great and typical periods of progress in the mental life of the normal child. They

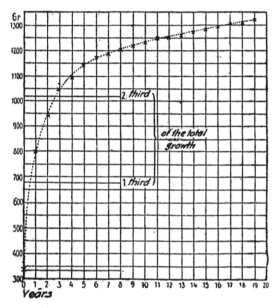

FIG. 6.—THE INCREASE IN THE WEIGHT OF THE BRAIN.

will not in each case be new paths and connections ; the finer structure of the individual centres themselves will probably also develop and differentiate. But we are as yet very far from having achieved this goal.

The increase in size of the brain cells and the development of the conducting systems is shown by a large increase in the weight of the brain. It is true, of course, that the growth of connective tissue partly accounts for this and in certain pathological cases there are quite different factors to be taken into consideration. The increase in weight of the brain is not by itself a satisfactory criterion of the mental development of the child, just as little as a particularly large brain in an adult necessarily points to particularly high mental achievements of its owner. Even the layman knows of hydrocephaly, and the pathology of the brain knows of other causes of high brain weight. It is only the typical average curve which can give us some valuable indications. In Fig. 6 we have such a curve, constructed from the data of Boyd. (The values of other authors are usually a little higher than those of Boyd. One can accept about 360 gms. as initial weight, 1,400 gms. as final weight in the case of boys; in the case of girls these weights are smaller by about 20 and 135 gms. respectively.)

We see from this curve that the weight of the brain is increased about fourfold in the course of development, at first growing very rapidly, afterwards more and more slowly. " *In the first three quarters of a year the brain doubles its initial weight, and trebles it before the end of the third year* " (Pfister). These facts are primarily to be connected with the perfecting of bodily movements, which probably takes the lion's share in that increase in weight. The general conclusions to be drawn from child psychology are also in complete agreement with this statement, for all the basic mental functions of the child are acquired in the first three or four years of its life and in its whole later life it does not make any more such fundamental progress as it does, for example, when it learns to speak. About the middle of the third decade the increase in weight of the brain stops, while the inner differentiation probably goes on; indeed, many are inclined to believe that a further increase in structural differentiation of the centres and neural paths is the basis of every new acquisition of knowledge and ability.

REFERENCES

H. FRIEDENTHAL, *Allgemeine und Spezielle Physiologie des Menschenwachstums*, 1914. (A rigorously scientific work with a special chemical theory of the processes of growth.)   C. H. STRATZ, *Der Körper des Kindes*, 3rd edn., 1909.   (For a wider circle, with many illustrations.) PH. BIEDERT, *Das kind, seine Körperliche und geistige Pflege von der Geburt bis zur Reife*, 2nd edn., by REIN and SELTER, 1911.   (Educational and School hygiene are in the foreground).—F. A. SCHMIDT, *Das Schulkind nach seiner Körperlichen Eigenart und Entwicklung*, 1914. (An excellent general exposition for teachers and school doctors.)

CHAPTER TWO

THE FIRST YEAR OF LIFE

5.—THE THREE LEVELS IN THE CHILD

(a). *Instinct.* The pathetic helplessness of new-born man is due to his *poverty in developed instincts.* The child *cries* in a state of *displeasure,* e.g. when its freedom of movement is restricted too much, or it is held into a cold bath. Further, the child *sucks and swallows* when taken to the breast, reacts differently to sweet, sour and bitter fluids that are introduced into its mouth   Finally, it possesses a few simple *protective reflexes,* such as closing the eyes when a bright light falls on them. This and similar simple reflexes, which can in principle be brought into action by every sense organ, is the whole stock of finished instincts which the child brings with it.[1] It does not follow from this, however, that all other instinctive actions are missing ; many of them only appear later. Man is born with certain elemental springs of action which keep life going ; in him, too, the higher life wells up out of the dark striving after existence, after activity, pleasure, happiness ; in him, too, certain fundamental lines of the life-plan are given from the beginning, only they are sketchy, undefined, highly in need of supplementing by training and intellect. Compared with the firmly regulated life of insects, the instincts of man appear muddled and disintegrated, even endowed with wide individual differences, so that we have to ask ourselves whether we are dealing with the same phenomenon in both cases.

[1] An accurate determination of all the modes of behaviour which the new-born babe and the somewhat older infant have at their disposal, will be found in : Ch. Bühler and H. Hetzer, " Inventar der Verhaltungsweisen des ersten Lebensjahres, in : *Soziologische und psychologische Studien über das erste Lebensjahr,* Jena, 1927.

Take as an example walking on two legs. Young fowls and ducks walk as soon as they creep out of the shell ; certain running birds (coursers) are so clever at balancing their bodies, that they can stand on one leg and scratch their heads with the other. All this they can do without previous practice. The human child has painfully to learn how to walk on two legs ; nevertheless, even here there is an instinct present, because, when its time has come, it strives of its own accord to get up and learns to sit and to stand. Once it can stand, the course of development drives it on. The rhythm of walking— alternately right-left— is so to speak, already present in the legs in a crude form, or rather in the brain, through which the legs are directed. True, the adults help it on, but that is not the important thing, for the child would also learn to walk without them. Suppose a child could grow up under conditions in which it never sees an upright, walking adult : I still believe that it will one day raise itself up and learn to walk. No doubt it will learn to do this a good deal later and more slowly than our own children ; but it will learn the same mode of propulsion quite of its own accord.

What, then, is the point of such a long apprenticeship ? Is it not a tremendous disadvantage, a set-back compared to the conditions in the fowl, which can walk and run immediately ? Now, in biology, we have to be very careful with purposive explanations, because they are, rightly, in bad repute since so much nonsense was talked about them in the 18th century. But in our case we are dealing with a general phenomenon, which challenges us to give an explanation, or, to express it more cautiously, which challenges us to think. Not only the use of its legs in walking, but also that of its hands in touching and grasping, even, within limits, looking around with its eyes have to be learnt by the human child. It seems to us that such far-reaching disadvantages compared with the animals must be dictated by some necessity, if we accept the theorem of the economy of nature, who like a good business man, usually only relinquishes small advantages where she can get bigger ones in exchange. The idea, that man has been able to achieve the extraordinary plasticity, i.e. educability, of his dispositions only by forgoing the fixity of the instincts, is not new. It has been said that the young fowl is able to walk on its two legs as soon as it is born, but for that it is unable to learn to climb, dance, or skate. This " for that " sounds plausible enough, but is nevertheless, as matters stand to-day, unprovable. One has only to think of the human tongue, which is capable of taking part in sucking and swallowing—a mechanism complete at birth—and yet is suitable for practising the extremely delicately differentiated and manifold movements of speaking.

One can observe human instincts in a very pure form in the lowest idiots, those unfortunate beings who are practically incapable of being trained in any way, so that they cannot even be taught not to defaecate in their rooms. When feeding-time comes round and the smell of food enters the nose, the mechanism of the food instinct is called into action : the nostrils quiver, the eyes are dilated and restlessness and excitement, even to sweating, take hold of the body ; the jaws begin to work, saliva collects in the mouth and flows out of the opened lips ; in short, it is the same spectacle that we are familiar with in dogs or in the animals at the zoo. The lowest idiots cannot feed themselves, or rather, cannot eat in human fashion with a spoon, but have to be fed. If one lets them have it, they greedily bolt double the quantity for a normal child of the same age and weight. When the doctors of lunatic asylums become more interested in psychology and investigate these phenomena from the point of view of the theory of levels, we shall soon be better informed about human instincts than we are to-day.

(b). *Training*. The first six months of life are almost entirely taken up by the acquisition of simple feats like grasping, sitting, crawling etc. Standing and walking follow a good deal later, and with the beginnings of language we shall be specially concerned. In all this, we repeat, instincts that gradually reach maturity are at work, as well as training, particularly self-training in play. All the other advances which the child makes during this time and beyond it, up to the last quarter of the first year, rest on the same basis. In this way a notable collection of special abilities is gradually acquired, enabling the small being to differentiate in its practical attitude towards repeatedly recurring events, persons, and things. The six months old infant, for instance, reacts differently towards its nurse than towards strangers, differently when it is approached with the bottle of milk or the bottle of medicine. In addition the adult makes use of language, to practise small artificial tricks—but of this more in the chapter on the understanding of language. In short : the child is a *trainable being*, like a clever dog, and nothing reveals to an external observer that it is soon to make rapid strides beyond the mental level of the dog.

The details of learning to look, grasp and walk have been thoroughly studied in the normal child and are well-known. In idiots, the higher we ascend, the more clearly do the characteristics of training appear. Indeed, we know of victims of mild mental deficiency who, in certain achievements of mechanical memory, apparently surpass the normal man, e.g. in remembering numbers and in mental arithmetic ; individuals, who can remember with the greatest ease hundreds of birthdates, addresses, numbers of trams or trains, etc., and reproduce them with the certainty of an automaton. This does not necessarily indicate a real superiority of memory, for as a rule their successes can be explained from the narrowing of their interests to a small, special field, together with years of practice in it. Under similar conditions the normal man can do as much, indeed far more. It would, of course, also be quite wrong to suspect the intelligence of a child which happens to be outstanding as regards the remembering of numbers.

(c). *Intellect.* I shall now describe when and how I

found the first achievements in a carefully observed child, from which intellect could be inferred. They were achievements of exactly the same type as those we are familiar with in chimpanzees (pp. 17, etc.), indeed there is a phase in the life of the child, which one might well designate the CHIMPANZEE-AGE. In the case of this particular child it was about the 10, 11 and 12th months. We see the termination of this age by progress in a new field, that of language, a step that is not taken by the chimpanzee, so far as we know. It is in the chimpanzee-age, therefore, that the child makes its first small discoveries. They are, of course, exceedingly primitive discoveries, but they are of the greatest importance for its mental development. We cannot proceed in our investigations in the same way as Köhler, because there is no question of dragging boxes about and climbing up them. Even the use of a stick transcends the skill of the child. But apart from this the child is also far more labile, one would like to say more unformed, than the 4 to 7-year old chimpanzees, who are almost fully grown at that age. Without knowing exactly what the salient features are, it will not be possible to discover the new element in the careless, random reactions of the child. Still, with the necessary patience and circumspection we shall also arrive at unequivocal results here.

We made use of the playful grasping of the child in devising experiments. At the age of nine months the child sits up in its bed and grasps at everything that comes within reach and attracts its attention, to take it to the mouth or to feel it. So we placed a piece of smooth wax cloth in front of the child and allowed it to grab, mostly at a piece of rusk. But there were always some difficulties which had to be overcome. For instance, a short, low glass plate was put between the rusk and the child, in order to see whether it would of itself try to get over or round the plate. Or the rusk was placed a little out of reach, while a piece of string attached to it was within reaching distance, to see whether the child would draw the rusk towards itself by means of the string. Or an ivory ring with which the child was wont to play, was passed over a bolt the thickness of a finger, fixed vertically to a board so that no amount of pulling or rattling would get the ring off : it had to be *lifted* off.

This ring experiment was also tried by Köhler on his chimpanzees. He found that it constitutes a very difficult problem which only the most gifted animals could definitely solve in their ' clearest ' moments.   We had the same experience with the child : it was only understood towards the middle of its second year that the ring had to be lifted off (without help, of course), but then it was also immediately able to take a key from a nail or a hat from a stick, besides lifting the ring off the bolt ; the child did not do this neatly and elegantly, it is true, but it certainly did so in a sensible fashion.   About this time the child also began to take great pleasure in playing with cardboard boxes, opening and closing them with unflagging interest, after it had been shown how to do this. The countess M. von Kuenburg has investigated the first attempts at abstraction by means of boxes of different colours, shapes and sizes, and has reported the results herself.

The experiment with the glass plate gave no definite result.   The child, soon after the commencement of the investigation, in its ninth month, reached round the plate in the correct way ; but we were unable to decide whether this was the result of training, or whether it was a discovery the child had made, because the solution often appeared to have been arrived at fortuitously after several attempts, knocking up against the plate with the hand, or groping round and along it.   It is possible that the child acted like the hen at the garden fence, or that the procedure only received a meaning later.

The experiments with the string and the biscuit, on the other hand, were more certain, but again it was not possible to fix the exact day on which the discovery had been made. At first, in its ninth month, the child regularly reached

E

out for the biscuit, taking no notice of the string. If this happened to come into its aimlessly grabbing hand, the child let go again or definitely pushed the string aside. Only during two sessions did it seem as though the connection between the two had been grasped, because several prompt solutions followed each other. Indeed I now believe that this was actually the case. But the next time everything had again been forgotten. It was only at the end of the tenth month that the child had completely mastered the situation. From now on we could place the string anywhere, for example on the extreme left, the biscuit being on the right, and the child would each time look about for the string and pull the biscuit towards itself, but only when the biscuit was too far away to be grasped directly. There were various reasons for discounting this as being merely the result of training. In the first place, these experiments had been carried out only once every few days and chance successes had been prevented, whereas for training both successes and numerous repetitions are necessary. Secondly, the characteristic transference to situations outside those of the actual experiment was in evidence, and thirdly we made the same observations that Köhler had made : One can at a glance recognize in the gestures of the child the difference between mechanically acquired and purposive action. Finally, during the eleventh month the child succeeded in a number of other manipulations, which gave one the impression that similar ' discoveries ' were involved. The most important one, however, that of language, was not made until the next month.

A repetition of these and similar experiments with other children is eminently desirable. The matter is of interest not merely because the appearance of intellect can here be objectively demonstrated for the first time, but for another, more general reason. The achievements of the chimpanzee are *quite independent of language* and in the case of man even in later life, technical thinking, or thinking in terms of tools, is far less closely bound up with language and concepts than other forms of thinking. It has been said that language is the prelude to the coming of man. That may be, but even before language comes the *thinking in terms of tools*, i.e. the realization of mechanical connections and the invention of mechanical means for mechanical ends. To put it briefly, before the advent of speech, action comes to have a *subjective meaning*, that is, it becomes consciously purposive.

REFERENCES

M. W. SHINN, *Notes on the Development of a Child* (California, 1893-9). K. W. DIX, *Körperliche und geistige Entwicklung eines Kindes*, 1. Heft : *Die Instinktbewegungen der ersten Kindheit*, 1911, 2. Heft : *Die Sinne*, 1912. E. u. G. SCUPIN, *Bubi im ersten bis dritten Lebensjahr*, 1903. The above-mentioned works draw their conclusions from careful observations on one and the same child over a long time. Their methods are different from those mentioned below. These works on the psychology of the sibling have reached their conclusions with the help of experimental and statistical methods. CH. BÜHLER, HETZER, HART, " Soziologische und psychologische Studien über das erste Lebensjahr," *Quellen und Studien zur Jugendkunde*, 5, Jena, 1927. CH. BÜHLER and LOTHAR SPIELMANN, " Die Entwicklung der Körperbeherrschung im ersten Lebensjahr," *Zeitschr. f. Psychol.*, CVII, (1928).

6.—THE FIRST STEPS IN THE DEVELOPMENT OF LANGUAGE

The beginnings of language are biologically older, and reach deeper down into the hierarchy of animals than the beginnings of thought. This is clear from the sounds animals produce. The clucking of a hen, for instance, is purely a matter of instinct, for when a chicken is hatched in an incubator and grows up without ever hearing the clucking of a hen, it will later nevertheless, emit precisely the same call as other hens . These sounds are inseparably built into the mechanism of the nursing instinct and show no variations that might indicate an adaptation of the individual to new situations, that is, point to training, much less to intellect. Other birds, such as parrots, can be trained to sounds and can learn to produce new combinations of sounds. The dog can learn to perform

different vocal expressions of his master. But in all
this no one has as yet been able to demonstrate traces of
intellect.

(a). *The sources.* The various sounds made by animals
are rightly looked upon as the biological foundation of
human language, which probably has its deepest roots in
the crying instinct of the child, an instinct functioning
copiously from the very first moment of its existence.
The *immediate* source of language in the child, however,
is not its cries, but its first *incoherent babbling*, an instinctive expression definitely distinguishable from crying.
From about its third month, the child produces these
sounds in moments of well-being. Just as it kicks its
legs and arms about, it playfully sets its vocal organs
going and soon derives so much pleasure from this
exercise that it keeps it up with great perseverance.
The result is that a number of different sounds soon make
their appearance, e.g. the r-like gurgling, when the
child is lying on its back and a drop of liquid collects in
its throat, aspirates, explosives produced by closing the
lips or the palate, and many others. Gradually clearer
and more constant complexes appear, such as ARRA,
MUMUM, BABA. Phonetics ought to register these sounds
with modern methods and analyse them, for they represent
the instinctive sound-material of all human languages, in
which as yet our children are indistinguishable from
Chinese, Eskimo or negro babies. Even children who are
born deaf begin to babble, which shows that the first
impulse is not derived from hearing other sounds. They
do not get very far with it, however, and this indicates
that in the case of the normal child, hearing soon plays an
important part.

The child derives pleasure from the acoustic phenomena
it produces; and therefore a motive for the endless
repetitions of the same movements of the vocal organs,
which have been somewhat grandly described as *babbling
monologues*. The psychologically important fact about
them is the formation of strong associations between the

auditory impression and the movements which produce it, for this is the essential basis of the later imitation of sounds the child hears, in which it has to translate what it has heard into vocal movements of its own. But for many months it is entirely self-dependent and forms ever new sound complexes through the pure joy of playing. It has only been possible to demonstrate definite imitations of what adults say to it, from about the middle of the first year. That is something new and is, of course, the beginning of the definite transformation of childish language into the languages of adults. At first the similarity of its imitations to the models is very small. The child has to deal with great difficulties even in the vocal combinations it produces spontaneously and therefore with even greater difficulties in the new ones. The gradual, imitative conquest of some hundreds of words, which go to form a colloquial modern language, is a tremendous achievement ; and every teacher knows that many children are still in the midst of this process of phonetic assimilation to the language of adults when they reach school-going age.

To go back for a moment : What is it that distinguishes childish babbling from crying ? In the first place, its greater *diversity*. All crying is not the same : It can be loud, rapidly or slowly changing, excited or phlegmatic, and there may be a few more shades. But if it were to be analysed phonetically, one would need but few signs to write it down. The case is entirely different with babbling. If everything that different children gradually produce spontaneously is brought together, it will be seen to comprehend the larger part of the acoustic qualities of all languages ; and beyond that it contains sounds which are not to be found in any of them. Here we have the source of the raw materials, the vocal stone-quarry, so to speak, of the human languages. More important, however, is a second distinction. The various cries are built into an instinctive mechanism, which serves the natural purpose of drawing the attention of the nurse to the child's needs. But the first babbling sounds that the child produces in play remain for a considerable time free from any meaning. They represent, as it were, property that has no master, which anyone may claim, or in our sense, to *which any meaning may be assigned*. That, as we shall soon see, is a very important fact. Though the first sounds of children of all races correspond, one and the same word never has quite the same import later on for any two children.

(*b*). *How does speech attain to meaning?* In the course of development, the understanding of language precedes its sensible expression. Several stages can be distinguished ; first the child begins to pay attention to spoken sounds, listens, when someone speaks, and shows pleasure at hearing the various sounds. At the second stage it turns towards the speaker as the source of sound. Thirdly, definite reactions are associated with definite sounds (words or series of words). Thus the child will turn towards the clock if you say TIC-TOC, or towards the mother, when someone says MAMA. There is also the sort of training no mother or nurse will forgo : How BIG IS MY BABY ? SAY PLEASE ! LET MAMA BITE ! These are achievements which can in no way be distinguished from animal training. It has been found that just as in the latter, the effects are sometimes brought about by the rhythm of the language used, or by some outstanding vowel. The child does not remain on this level for long, but soon reaches understanding in the narrower sense of the term. *Gestures* are a great help towards this. One can observe how, quite early, about the middle of the first year or even sooner, the child is differently affected by a cheerful, smiling face than by a sad or angry one, and some months later it goes so far as to cry when it sees someone else cry. It may be that instinctive factors play a part in the transmission of gestures ; at any rate it is through the facial expressions that the first reflections of the speaker's state of mind are cast into the child's soul.

It is at this stage in our study of the understanding of language, during the last quarter of the first year or a little later, that the supremely important *first words which make sense are spoken by the child itself.* They are ' babbled ' words like MAMAM, NANA, DADA, etc., or reduplicated words like DEDDA for Bertha, TIT-TIT for tic-toc (clock), which the child tries to repeat after the grown-ups. What is the meaning of such words ? That can be determined from their use on different occasions. For example, the son of Preyer on the first anniversary of his birth got hold of the word ' *Geburtstag,*' (birthday), eagerly repeated it as *burtsa* and from then on this word always appeared when the child was pleased with anything. It was thus a kind of joyous exclamation, a ' shout of delight.' This is typical, for *the first sensible words are either such affective expressions, or the signs of some wish.* When the child says MAMA, it is either expressing some affect connected with the mother, or it wants something from her, when it says CHAIR, something exciting has happened in connection with it, or the child wants to be put on the chair.

Let us stop here for a moment. Up to this point we are unable to find anything in the child's language, which could not, in principle, appear in any animal. The sounds themselves have nothing specifically human about them ; their combinations may seem to have, but even these any well-trained parrot will bring forth just as well as the one-year-old. Nor is the meaning of these sounds specifically human, for even in the dog affects and desires are expressed by differentiated series of sounds ; they are different in pleasure, anger, fear, or when it ' begs.' Let us conceptualize this : when a sound or other sign, e.g. a gesture, exists or is suited to the purpose of betraying, or indicating, some psychic state of the individual making this sound or sign, we shall call this the FUNCTION OF INDICATION. When a sound exists or is suitable for releasing in the audience a certain attitude, we shall call this the FUNCTION OF

RELEASE. The clucking of the hen, for example, obviously fulfils the natural purpose of making the chicks run to the mother, or at least of keeping them together. The so called warning cry of many gregarious animals that place ' sentinels ' like the chamois, belongs to this category. When the particularly observant ' sentinel ' notices something suspicious, he emits a cry and the whole herd takes to flight. That is release. Whether the animal itself knows anything about the objectively purposive connection or not, is for the time being irrelevant to our concept.

The functions of indication and release are common to human language and the cries and calls of animals. Indication and release, the biologically oldest natural aids of sounds that are similar to language, are also the first to appear when the babbling of children comes to have a meaning. But human language has a third fundamental function, which has not as yet been demonstrated in any animal. I call this the REPRESENTATIONAL FUNCTION. Any sentence from a scientific work may serve to make this clear, for example the sentence, " London is situated on the Thames." What does this sentence do in a book on geography ? It obviously enables us to infer a certain fact, something which a map might do equally well. That Cologne Cathedral has two towers, I could ' read off ' from a photograph instead of from a sentence, just as I could ' read off ' from a graph that the fever rose to 104.9⁰ in the evening. To summarize : geographical maps, photographs and curves are *means of representing* objects and propositions, each in its own way. But the most general and most important method of representation which the human mind has created is language.

(c). *The discovery of the naming function.* The first book of Genesis tells us how God brought all the animals in Paradise to Adam, who gave them each a name. The invention of names was, if not the first, certainly one of the most important steps in the history of the mental evolution of mankind. Every one of our children has to

take it again. This usually happens at about the end
of the first year, the beginning of the second year, or
a little later. The first noteworthy phenomenon is that
the principle of the invariability of objects establishes
itself in the use of words, the second is the beginning of
the *questions as to names* and the third a *sudden, rapid
increase of vocabulary.* In explaining these, we must
start with the phenomenon of the questions as to names,
because this is the most important. When new objects
force themselves on the attention of the child, it expresses
a wish in the form of unmistakable gestures, or by means
of words spoken in a questioning tone (e.g., that ? What's
that ?). This wish the person who is asked can satisfy
by pronouncing some word. As a rule an adult will
correctly interpret the situation, pronounce the word as
carefully as possible and repeat it several times ; the
child will listen attentively and try to imitate the word.
What is going on here ?

The constant expression of the same wish and the
peculiar way of satisfying it, both need explanation.
One can say that the child now has a general tendency,
when attentively perceiving an object, to say a word,
not just any word, but some definite word every time.
On the basis of already existing reproductive associations
it pronounces the word ' dada ' when it sees the father and
the corresponding associated words for other objects ;
it is only when an object is met with that has not as yet
been associated with anything, that the child stops and
calls for the help of the adults by means of unequivocal
gestures. This shows that the situation calls up a ' problem ' in the child's mind, a problem for which it has the
general scheme of solution—enunciating a word—but
not always the particular means—a definite word.
Sometimes a familiar word comes up as substitute,
as when a town child reacts with wowwow on seeing a
calf or even calls a cow wowow. This is the same kind
of situation as that of the chimpanzee when he needs a
stick and grasps at objects which would otherwise not

appear to him as sticks at all (cf. p. 11). Incidentally, as Köhler has reported, the chimpanzee also takes the easier way of ' appealing for help ' to a person standing near.

That the child should regularly take up this attitude is, psychologically, the most remarkable aspect of the matter. It proves, no more and no less, that one of the most important discoveries (inventions) of man has penetrated into his mind, the fact *that everything has a name.* Look at it from whatever side you will, at the decisive point a psychological parallel to the discoveries of the chimpanzee will appear. That general effect of which we spoke on p. 14—the transference of a few cases to all—forces itself on our attention. In view of the observations we have made in the preceding paragraph on the ' chimpanzee-age, of the child, we cannot as yet expect to see the characteristics of suddenness and ' once and for all ' manifested quite as clearly in its case. On the other hand, both these aspects appear as clearly as we could wish in a report on the blind and deaf child Helen Keller, who only made this discovery in her seventh year. It was two months since her teacher, Miss Sullivan, had started instructing her in the finger alphabet. She writes : " We went out to the pump-house, and I made Helen hold her mug under the spout while I pumped. As the cold water gushed forth, filling the mug, I spelled ' w-a-t-e-r, in Helen's free hand. The word coming so close upon the sensation of cold water rushing over her hand seemed to startle her. She dropped the mug and stood as one transfixed. A new light came into her face. She spelled ' water ' several times. Then she dropped on the ground and asked for its name and pointed to the pump and the trellis, and suddenly turning round she asked for my name. . . . All the way back to the house she was highly excited, and learned the name of every object she touched, so that in a few hours she had added thirty new words to her vocabulary."[1] I must admit that this

[1] Helen Keller, *The Story of My Life,* New York, 1903, p. 316.

report seems to me a little dramatized. I have myself followed the teaching of several deaf and dumb children and have made enquiries about other cases from reliable teachers, but have never found that it was possible to date the occurrence of the decisive step to a second. The course of development rather followed those minor discoveries we have described in the preceding paragraph. Perhaps that experience at the well was only the final act of a long process. However that may be—and Helen Keller actually was an exceptionally active child, mentally, and had lost her sight and hearing relatively late—there is certainly no psychological impossibility in Miss Sullivan's description, and, what is for us the main consideration, in principle every child goes through the same experience, even if somewhat more slowly.

We break off here, to take up the development of language in Chapter Six.

REFERENCES

W. AMENT, *Die Entwicklung von Sprechen und Denken beim Kinde*, 1899. E. MEUMANN, *Die Entstehung der ersten Wortbedeutungen beim Kinde*, 1902. CL. and W. STERN, *Die Kindersprache*, 1907. (This gives further references.) 4th edn., 1928.

7.—THE NATURE OF THE CONSCIOUS STATES OF THE INFANT

We cannot decide with certainty whether the new-born child already experiences pain and pleasure, whether it has some other primitive form of consciousness or not. In interpreting psychologically the various movements and reactions it carries out, we must proceed with extreme care. The famous clinician Kussmaul and others have dropped fluids of different tastes and at body temperature on the tongue of new-born infants by means of a fine brush, so that the disturbing influence of warmth and touch reflexes was avoided. In this way they obtained pure and quite characteristic taste reactions. It was found that sugar-water releases the swallowing

mechanism and gives the face the expression for
'sweetness,' whereas bitter and sour liquids were not
swallowed, but were either actively ejected from the
mouth, or passively allowed to flow out again. The
facial expression for 'sourness' could be distinguished
from that of 'bitterness' by the corners of the mouth,
which were drawn down in the former case. What
follows from this ? Surely it means no more than that
the sensory mechanism of the taste sense, that is the
taste-buds in the tongue and their nervous system, is
already functioning, as far as it is needed for reflexes.
It is questionable whether the nervous impulses are at
this stage conducted as far as those areas of the cortex
in which the sensations of taste arise. Anatomically
these parts of the cortex are ready to function at birth.
But observations of children born without a cortex, who
are no different from normal children during the first
few days, at any rate as far as the broader manifestations
of life are concerned, would seem to indicate that the
cortex does not function at once. It is quite possible
that the new-born child is a pure 'spinal being,' of whose
central nervous system only the spinal cord and those
parts of the brain belonging functionally to the spinal
cord are active. We have no material for imagining
how such a being ' feels.'

In the first months after birth the various sensory and
motor centres of the cortex one after another become
active and ready for functioning, but even from this fact
we can draw no conclusions as to the states of consciousness of the infant. One has to fall back on the reactions
observed in the living child. Naïve mothers see in the
first smile, which usually appears about three weeks after
birth, a certain sign of awaking 'humanity,' without
knowing that it also appears in animals, e.g., apes. The
whole first quarter is traditionally called the 'silly'
quarter, the opinion being, apparently, that only after
this can we see any sign of human 'intelligence.' Well,
in the sense in which we naïvely talk of stupid and

intelligent dogs, that is dogs which learn easily and those which do not, this may be allowed to pass if we bear in mind what has been discussed above. At any rate, during the whole of the chimpanzee-age of the child (cf. p. 48), there is no evidence that it has more numerous or more differentiated conscious processes than other trainable beings.

At this point the attempt at a more exact scientific interpretation comes up against a serious lacuna in our knowledge. In a word, we do not know what the *biological functions of consciousness* are. In order to determine what conscious processes are linked up with some specific, objectively determinable achievement, we must know in general why consciousness exists, why it is necessary. Nature does not create superfluous institutions on a large scale. If the mechanism of in-stinctive actions runs just as smoothly and exactly without consciousness in bees and ants as it would if strivings and feelings were also present, then there is no scientific ground for ascribing consciousness to them ; and if in the individual simple kinds of adaptation to special conditions are brought about by training, these will result without help from consciousness. If someone has had an attack of scarlet fever or typhus, his organism is permanently, or for a long time, protected against attacks of that kind by very effective arrangements of which he does not ' feel ' or ' know ' anything. On the other hand we may retain a conscious revulsion for some foods which made us ill. Would the same protection in this case be possible without consciousness ? Or think again of the hen and the garden fence ! If an effective reaction is to be built up by training, a definite association between clear sense-impressions and a single mode of behaviour must crystallize from the random changes of behaviour. Are there perhaps phases in this process in which some form of consciousness is able to give help unobtainable otherwise ? We speak of the pleasure of success and the displeasure of failure and it may be that truly conscious processes are to be understood by this. Besides, what are we to understand by ' clear sense-impressions ' ? Whether the hole in the fence is a little larger or smaller, whether, seen from different distances, it gives rise—in an absolute sense—to larger or smaller retinal pictures, all this should be irrelevant to the argument. Perhaps this is only possible because the hen already has ' impressions of complexes,' or perceives general configurations. This would be a faculty of consciousness that could hardly be replaced by a mechanical equivalent. But enough of conjectures ; they were only meant to point out the directions in which we are to seek explanations. It is even possible that the first conscious processes reach further down still, into the realm of instincts. In the case of the child our interpretations will become more reliable, the more closely his achievements approximate to those of adults.

Thoughtful mothers may perhaps express doubts about our views. Those who have had the opportunity of observing children from the first moment of their existence, know that certain differences in character appear from the very first. One child eagerly took to the breast, another gently ; one had a tendency to explosive crying, another patiently allowed anything to be done to it ; one was ' clumsy ' and difficult to teach, so that it could only be persuaded with much trouble to suck properly at the breast or bottle, while another was good at it immediately, etc. I do not doubt that such differences in the nature of children can appear from the very first day, but it has nothing to do with our question. For such differences are also observed in animals. They are probably founded prior to all consciousness in the unknown hereditary qualities of the individual and are not bound up with conscious processes.

CHAPTER THREE

THE DEVELOPMENT OF THE PERCEPTIONS
OF THE CHILD

CERTAIN spiders that rush out of their tubular nest with machine-like regularity every time a fly gets into their net, killing the fly and dragging it in to be sucked dry, sometimes behave quite differently when a living fly is set down before them. They retreat from this fly as from an enemy and take up a fighting posture. It is said that the hungry spider will not bite even when the fly, in trying to escape, comes into contact with its talons or jaws.[1] If this were always the case, we should say: A perfect example of the fact, that with instincts as with mechanical automata, the exact conditions for which they have been constructed must be realized. The hunting method of the spider has been laid down once and for all, and in it the catching of its prey inside the nest has not been provided for. The question then arises, why should the mechanism of the predatory instinct sometimes fail in the nest? Is it because certain antecedents are missing that the spider does not bite, just as in an automatic machine the coin has to fall down before the lever of the chocolate drawer works? Or is the simultaneous complex of impressions that the spider receives from a fly struggling in the web different to the one it receives inside the nest and therefore ineffective? We have an analogy to the latter state of affairs in the combination lock of a safe.

The second possibility raises the problem whether the spider is incapable of appreciating single objects, such as we ourselves are familiar with. Perhaps the struggling

---

[1] H. Volkelt, " Uber die Vorstellungen der Tiere," *Arbeiten zur Entwicklungs psychologie.* (2. Heft), 1914.

63

object in the nest acts differently on the spider to the struggling object in the web, because the spider is not able to isolate and comprehend some of the component parts of the whole complex of impressions as that thing we humans call a fly. It may be that in the very primitive consciousness of the lower animals there is as yet no differentiation of impressions into isolated objects. The development of the perceptions of the child may also pass through such a primitive stage. Possibly that is so, but no empirical grounds for this assumption are known. One would have to carry out similar experiments on infants, that is, investigate more closely the behaviour of the young child in usual and unusual situations, to see whether after a small or a larger change it will similarly fail to recognize objects, because they are not sufficiently isolated from their surroundings. The observations of Volkelt have been challenged. More recent investigations have at least shown that it cannot be regarded as the rule that the garden spider fails to recognise its prey inside the tubular nest. On the contrary, the behaviour of these spiders has proved on closer examination to be unexpectedly variable and adaptable. This makes invalid the assumption, that there is something *radically* lacking in the sphere of perceptions. It is another question whether, after all, some of the remaining facts can not be interpreted in terms of our hypothesis. Even if the capacity to isolate impressions is present, it need not be as highly developed as it is in man. Moreover, as far as the obvious difference between instinct and training is concerned, this will naturally be affected by showing that here or there training goes deeper than was originally assumed. The residue of instinctive and automatic factors in the behaviour of spiders still remains large enough.[1]

---

[1] Cf. F. Baltzer, " Beiträge zur Sinnesphysiologie und Psychologie der Webespinnen." *Mitteilungen d. Naturforsch. Ges. in Bern*, 1923, (Heft 10). R. Demoll, " Über die Vorstellungen der Tiere," *Zool. Jahrb.* xxxviii (1921), *Abt. f. allg. Zool.* J. A. Bierens de Haan, " Sur les représentations des animaux," *Arch. d. Psych.* xviii (1922).

One thing, however, is certain : the higher trainable animals, like the dog, can be trained to react single 'objects' that have to be comprehended in isolation. Furthermore, it is certain that the child attains very early to the perception of objects, for no sooner can it grasp with some sureness, than it recognizably busies itself with isolated objects as such. Occasionally coloured spots, no larger than the head of a fly, attract the child's attention and stimulate it to grasp at them ; often, indeed, this isolating of single objects from their spatial surroundings and their recognition as such goes much further than with adults. The child in later years has to relearn how to interpret the impression of the whole and take account of complex properties, or, metaphorically speaking, not to overlook the wood for trees. At this time, too, the principle of the invariability of objects becomes objectively demonstrable in the discovery of the naming function (cf. p. 56).

Let us turn from these general questions to a closer analysis of the child's perceptions. The perceptions of adults are complicated events, which, apart from the processes of sensation, involve memory and a number of other intellectual functions. Indeed, we can say without undue exaggeration, that a great part of our thinking takes place in the perceptions and their immediate con-comitants. " It is seeing that makes an artist " ; to be able to perceive, assimilate and observe is the essential a b c of philosophy or science. How does the child learn to perceive ? To make his communication with the outside world possible, the infant brings with him well-developed sense-organs that are ready to function, so that it can not be a case of developing the sense organs themselves, or their specific functions (receiving impres-sions and transmitting the resultant excitation to the nerves leading to the brain). We find the idea expressed now and then—for instance in investigations on the colour sense of the child—that this is not so. To keep to this example, it is said that the eye is originally merely

F

a photographic apparatus capable of differentiating only between light and shade. In the course of the first months or years it can only register the wealth of colours physiologically. But this is an error, due to insufficient knowledge of the anatomical and physiological conditions. No, what do develop in perceptions can in the main be only the processes of psychic ' assimilation ' of impressions, the processes by which finer appreciations of space and time, attention and abstraction, comprehension of shape, number and relation are achieved. Let us investigate them in order.

8.—THE DEVELOPMENT OF THE PERCEPTION OF SPACE AND TIME

(a) *The appreciation of depth.* Helmholtz writes in his *Physiological Optics :* " I can remember as a child passing by the spire of the garrison church in Potsdam and seeing people on the balustrade, whom I took to be dolls. I asked my mother to take them down for me, believing she could do this by merely reaching up with her hands. I remember the incident so well, because it was this mistake which taught me the law of perspective, that is, the diminution of size with distance." The age is not stated. It happened, at a guess, in the third, fourth, or fifth year. In the same way still younger children on the mother's arm may demand the moon from heaven. This is not to be wondered at, for even we adults do not see the moon and stars at an infinite distance, but at a finite one, fixed to a blue dome called the sky, further away than the arm can reach, it is true, but not more than a few miles. If an inhabitant of the plains goes into the mountains for the first time, he is apt to underestimate the distances between summits very much, as well as their distances from him, but when he walks there himself, the panorama becomes wider and deeper to his perceptions.

Our impression of great distances is therefore the result of our own experience, our conception of the world (in the original sense of the word) broadens, when we pace out its distances ourselves. So we can assume that the further we go back in childhood, the narrower the world must have seemed. A child of six months has only mastered, by its movements, that part of space which lies within its grasp ; before that, i.e., before it can sit up and reach out after things, it is able to get only a few spatial experiences, e.g., by moving its head when put to the breast, and later on by licking and touching objects that reach its mouth. Three stages have therefore been distinguished : *mouth-space, touch-space* and *distant-space*. Is there anything in this ? The idea is quite useful for indicating a preliminary line of investigation, but it has not as yet stood the test of observed facts. The matter is certainly more complex. Reaching for the moon or other distant objects is not the general rule at the ' grasping-space ' stage. Binocular vision, which gives us immediate and unmistakable criteria of depth, is involved, as well as other factors. Some competent experimenter ought to take up the problem afresh.

(*b*) *Nativism in the perception of space.* The plain fact that adults cannot experience colours and qualities of touch otherwise than as extended and localized in some particular spot, whilst this does not necessarily seem to be the case for sounds and smells, has given rise to much speculative ingenuity and to the so-called ' genetic ' or ' empirical ' views on the origin of the perception of space. That is to say, our consciousness of the extensity and order of objects in space is supposed to be not something inherent, but something that appears during the course of the mental development of the individual. The first question that arises is whether consciousness without spatial perception is thinkable at all. *Distinguo*, I distinguish : if one tries to imagine a position in which one has sense impressions without any spatial data at

all, one's efforts of abstractive imagination will be in vain.
On the other hand it is quite easy to ' think ' away the
perception of space. We can think four or *n*-dimensional
space, but no one can conceive it ; can we not then be
conscious of the wealth of sensory qualities and their
gradations of intensity without extensity and localization ? The famous theory of Lotze, that the spatial
data are only developed later, was therefore rightly
taken seriously even by his opponents. But it seems to
me nevertheless possible to refute it by considerations of
a general psychological nature, without reference to
particular facts of mental development.

Even if he cannot refute it completely, the psychologist
can at least show what proof for its justification he
demands—a proof which it will probably not be possible
to give. My considerations are the following : nothing
can come out of nothing ; this is the principal premise
from which Lotze also starts. The ordering of sense
data into left and right, down and up, back and front,
must therefore in some way be pre-established in the
sense data themselves. Lotze, however, assumes that
this order originally has the character of a *qualitative
manifold*. Just as sounds can be arranged in order of
pitch, or colours in the order of their colour tone (red—
orange—yellow, etc.), so he assumes that the impressions
of the sense of sight or touch have ' qualities of neigh-
bourhood.' That is, they have distinctive signs, and the
whole local arrangements of the sensory points of our
skin is a systematic copy of these. Can one conceive
that by associations, fusions, or in any other way, a series
of similar qualities can be transformed into one of spatial
localities, such as the points on a straight line represent ?
In the natural sciences that employ measurement, purely
qualitative determinations and differences are avoided,
for the simple reason that one cannot *measure* them.
Can it be, then, that the spatial perceptions, the sphere
to which measurements are essentially germane, have
proceeded by ' experience ' from a perception of purely

qualitative order ? This seems to me hardly less para-
doxical than the contention that, say, colours have
originated from smells or sounds from sensations of
pressure. One can conceive of the distance between
two points being subdivided *ad libitum*, but not the
distance (difference) between two qualities. If there is
a characteristic distinction between them, it is hard to
see how one can have ' developed ' from the other.[1]

Theoretically there is hardly much more to be said
for the less radical view that a vague kind of ' planeness '
is the primary basis of space perception (primary, because
it is inherent in the nature of visual and touch impressions), and that depth—the third dimension—is something new added by experience. As against this, we may
say that in developed consciousness we can find no
difference between the perception of depth and the perception of height and breadth. Above all, it is not
conceivable how such a plane can exist in consciousness
without the awareness of distance from the eye (or more
correctly, from the starting point of the directions of
vision) and without the awareness of behind and before.
The idea of development does not seem to me to call for
such forced hypotheses. We can conceive of organisms
which move adequately in three-dimensional space without consciousness at all, merely with the help of a physiological reaction mechanism adapted to this end. But
if for some reason the necessity for being conscious of
space arises, this will probably not develop out of other,
already present factors in consciousness. It will only
develop in close collaboration with such factors and will
contain within itself from the beginning the capacity
for appreciating three-dimensionality, however imper-
fectly. More we cannot say at present.

(c) *The differentiation of the principal directions.* Even
now the field for investigation in the child remains wide
and rich enough, for it is self-evident that the child's

---

[1] More detail in : Bühler, article on " Zeitsinn und Raumsinn,"
Handwörterbuch d. Naturwissenschaften, Vol. x, (1915).

perception of space does not immediately attain the accuracy of which the practised architect or artist is capable and is not equipped with the conceptual clarity of the mathematician. The question as to how the principal directions of visual space, *vertical* and *horizontal*, attain to their pre-eminent importance, leads to interesting problems. The vertical forces itself upon us as the direction of the earth's attraction, that is, through the pressure sense of the skin and the muscular sense. That we even remain orientated about above and below when diving under water, is due to the functioning of another sense organ, the static apparatus in the interior of the head. It would be interesting to know how the four different sense organs—those of pressure, effort, sight and the static apparatus—learn to co-operate with each other in the very young child.

The differentiation between *right* and *left* belongs to another category of facts. During the course of the second year, i.e., long before the names right and left are properly understood and applied, the practical preference of one hand over the other makes its appearance. The vast majority of children becomes right-handed, but even at this age some 2 to 4 per cent. reveal themselves as left-handed. For the disposition to right or left-handedness is hereditary and not in any way acquired, though the statistical material is as yet too sparse to enable us to understand the laws by which it is transmitted. It was at first supposed that it followed the simplest form of the Mendelian rules and that left-handedness is recessive. As in the case of blue eyes, two left-handed parents could therefore only have left-handed children (cf p. 22). Observations on the rare cases in which both parents are left-handed would be most welcome at this stage ; the matter does not seem to be quite as simple, judging by the few cases which have come under my notice.

The anatomical bases for the preference of one half of the body over the other are to be sought for in the cortex.

It has long been known that the functions of speech are localised on one side of the cortex, the left in the case of a right-handed person, and vice versa ; but in accordance with newer findings, this has to be modified in an essential point : the centre for the speech impulses does not lie exclusively on the right or left ; there is a corresponding centre on the other side and it is only the *finest efforts*, the most delicate regulations and co-ordinations that are dealt with by one side only. Only the highest authorities in the system of offices dealing with the movements of speech are housed on one side, as it were. The same is true of all the one-sided finer manipulations such as writing, drawing, etc. From this we must draw an important conclusion for school practice. A left-hander can be forced to write and draw with his right hand and he will make some progress up to a certain point ; but in this way he will not realize the highest that lies in his capacity, because the faculties of the preferred half of the brain lie idle. Bimanual practice, which was in fashion for a time, is therefore also unable to satisfy certain exaggerated hopes placed in it, a result, by the way, which has been verified by extensive experiments.

(d) *The idea of time.* The span of durations which we can clearly grasp and compare with each other, is not longer than a few seconds. In the ' empty ' intervals between taps for instance, it is at most five seconds long. Above that one has to count or use other helps. The consciousness of the flux and duration of events that we have ourselves experienced, or are reliving in imagination, and which have occupied hours, days or years, can therefore not be called clear representation in the sense in which we can have a clear, conscious representation of moderately large spaces. Substitutes, such as spatial distances or other conceptual schemata, take their place. When the child learns to repeat short and long syllables correctly and to sing or otherwise to imitate simple rhythms, it must be able to appreciate short durations. It would pay, and would probably not be too difficult, to examine this more accurately experimentally. The differential and symbolic appreciation of longer durations, on the other hand, will most likely be acquired very late, since the child cannot count or otherwise fix easily recognizable marks in a monotonous series of events. Two cases have to be distinguished : *times of expectation* and *remembered times*. To give an example : an object in uniform motion disappears behind a screen. It is required to determine beforehand the exact moment at which it will reappear on the other side. If I am not mistaken, we already find something which is similar to this in hunting animals. Of the child we know that expectation is already shown during the first year.[1]

In another case, something has happened seconds, minutes, hours ago. How long ago is it ? Until a remarkably late age the child lacks useful standards for such judgments. The majority of six-year-olds has as yet no clear idea of the meaning of words like minute, hour, week, month. It is not known whether this is due merely to the arithmetical nature of the concepts and whether it would be any better if we still used the length of a *pater noster* or similar methods of practical life, or whether we are dealing with special difficulties in the appreciation of duration.

The *temporal order* of events is determined either by the continuous ' now,' the experienced present, or by one of the members of the series itself. I do not know what the circumstances are in the most primitive peoples ; it seems to me that comparative philology ought to have occasion to enquire into this. The child probably realizes of its own accord that there is an order in regular, daily, repeated series of events. Later on it understands the series of the principal times of the day. The physiological basis for this is given by the mechanism of association. When one thing after another enters the conceptual world of the child, as in games involving memory or expectation, consciousness of temporal succession will

---

[1] Ch. Bühler, *Kindheit und Jugend*, pp. 20 *et seq.*

not necessarily be present from the very beginning. In any case the child cannot pay attention to more than three things at a time, because its appreciation of groups is limited (cf. p. 79). But we may accept the fact, that the understanding of ' before ' and ' after ' (originally perhaps acquired in perceptual situations) is practised by playing games which require various things to be associated. In such games temporal succession is contained as an ordering principle. By introducing disturbing factors into such fixed, memorized series in some ingenious fashion, it may become possible to create experimental conditions that will enable us to follow the development of this understanding.

The theory of the conception of time is as yet full of riddles ; but nothing is more difficult to understand than the plain fact of the flowing ' now.' Theoretically this is a point, and therefore without duration. The ' now ' is at the root of every adequate and immediate concept of time ; it is that point at which past and future must somehow meet in order to come into our consciousness. In reality, what we experience as the present has duration, just as any seen or touched ' point ' has extensity. The experienced present is in principle no more than the point at which the large spans of past and future are projected. But this in no sense exhausts the facts. In our imagination we also project from temporal points of the actual past and the actual future. But let us return to the child. I quote an observation which Cl. and W. Stern made on their daughter at the age of 5 ; 1. During an imaginary game she writes to her absent father about what is happening to-day. She explains orally that when the father will receive the letter to-morrow he will already know that this will then have been yesterday and proceeds to describe the events as though the letter had been read. This is a considerable achievement for such a young child. When the words *to-day, to-morrow, yesterday*, etc., appear in the vocabulary of the child, as usually happens about the middle of the third year, sometimes a little earlier, sometimes later, they point to something temporal, it is true, but they are often applied in any order ; e.g., *we went for a walk to-morrow,* or *we shall do this yesterday.* As a rule at this stage the first distinction is made between past and present as such. If the child is consoled by being promised the fulfilment of a wish on the morrow, this does not mean anything more definite to him than ' next week ' or ' next year ' or ' when you have grown up.' Since such events affect the child very intimately, it will be readily understood that the emotionally coloured ' to-morrow ' is regularly used several months before ' yesterday.' At least a year passes before the child realizes at all clearly that each to-morrow becomes a to-day, and each to-day a yesterday. It is usual to explain the meaning of the terms ' day-after-to-morrow ' and those for still more remote points of time by counting the number of nights which have to pass : " *you must sleep once, twice . . . more.*" This will really be the best explanation of such terms, first, because the child cannot count far, and secondly, because it is very difficult to find suitable objects that the child can count in its imagination.

Very important problems of general interest are therefore involved in the development of the perception of time, the (symbolic) idea of time and the concept of time. What is lacking above all is a theoretical analysis of the concept of time.

REFERENCE :

W. STERN, "Die Entwicklung des Raumbewusstseins in der ersten Kindheit," *Zeitschr. f. angew. Psych.* II (1909).

9.—THE PERCEPTION OF SIZE, SHAPE, AND NUMBER

Some things are recognised by some of their sensory qualities and take their name from them, as, for example, the sorrel and the chestnut get their names from their colour. We shall discuss this in the next chapter. The giant and the dwarf are defined by means of their great or small size ; the sphere by its form ; the troika, the bicycle and the quadruped by a certain number of their component parts. There can be no doubt that sizes and shapes become important in the perceptions of a child at a very early age. Let us discuss this in detail.

(a) *Size.* The capacity for appreciating sizes is developed to a high degree of perfection in the first three years. Binet has performed experiments to test this on his $2\frac{1}{2}$ and 4 year old children. He placed before them straight lines drawn on paper and asked them which was longer, which shorter. Even the younger girl understood what was to be done and was able to distinguish differences of one-twentieth without hesitation, and without thinking about the matter she immediately pointed each time to the longer line and said, " That is the biggest," then to the other, saying, " That is the smallest." It was no good waiting, if she did not judge at once. She was unable to compare the lines when they were shown in succession. Under similar conditions adults are capable of appreciating differences four to five times as small ($1/80$ to $1/100$), i.e., two lines are distinguishable as different when one is 80, the other just 81 millimetres or centimetres long. The elder girl was also able to compare angles with almost the same exactness attained by untrained adults. It is desirable to know what the attitude of the children would be to exceptionally large and exceptionally small distances, and further, how accurately they would be able to compare magnitudes that are at different distances from them. Within certain limits, adults perceive the sizes of objects independently of their relative distances. For instance, I can easily compare correctly a book within reaching distance, with one several yards away on the shelf. Expressed differently : the visual angle under which objects are seen is not the only factor determining the impression we have of its size ; by means of a process not yet fully understood, the distance is always taken into account as well. We have recently found that this is true to a remarkable degree for the perceptions of a child of two, although it is, naturally, subject to the law of practice. It has been found that there is a gradual progress in this field up to the age of ten.[1]

(b) *Shape.* Various experiences of everyday life go to show that the child recognises certain things by their shape even in its first year. A useful method for investigating this at such an early age has however not yet been developed. Later, when the child begins to name objects, we can give it pictures and drawings to interpret. It was found that pictures in books, photographs, and outline drawings are interpreted surprisingly well as early as the second year. At the age of 1; 1 Shinn's niece, for instance, could pick out her father in a photograph of a group of nine. Stern has shown that this depends mainly on *outlines.* He drew simple outlines on a board in front of a child aged 1; 10, whilst it anxiously waited to see what was coming next. Very few characteristic lines sufficed to enable it to name correctly a chair, table, dog, horse, man, etc. This is of general psychological interest and of great importance for the later drawings of the child itself.

The ancients have reported of more than one renowned painter, that he had represented ripe grapes so naturally, that even birds were misled into pecking at them. This in no sense proves that animals 'understand' pictures, but rather the contrary, since they are incapable of distinguishing pictures from real objects under the given conditions. Now it is remarkable that we can clearly distinguish three stages in the development of pictorial appreciation in young children.[2] At first, pictures are nothing more to the child than bits of coloured paper that it can grasp and tear up. Then it begins to recognise what is represented by the picture and treats the pictures

---

[1] Cf. Franz Beyrl, " Über die Grössenauffassung bei Kindern," *Z. Ps.*, c (1926).
[2] Major, *First Steps in Mental Growth*, p. 251 *et seq.*

of objects just like the objects themselves. It is only in a third phase that it makes a practical distinction between a picture and reality. During the second stage, for instance, a child was just as frightened at a picture of a cat as at the cat itself, and could not be persuaded to touch it. Another child wanted to touch the eyes of people in photographs in the same way in which it was for a time accustomed to touch those of real people, and so on.[1] In my opinion we have to distinguish two different moments in the progress which leads to the third stage. In the *first* place the child originally grasps at any spots of light or shade on the floor and through repeated failure learns to distinguish these plane and fleeting objects of vision from the solid and unchanging ones. In the same way it will learn to manipulate the sheets of paper on which pictures are drawn in a different way to real objects. This will be applied to the represented figures, which, for a time, may still be interpreted as real ones. The second step is the dawning of the supremely important realization that pictures have a *representational function*. E. Wiehemeyer has recently made some experiments on the connection between the acquisition of the naming function in language and the recognition of pictures. He was able to test the ability of the child to recognise pictures independently of its ability to name them. The usual procedure up till then had been to show the child the picture and get it to name the picture. It was shown that only children who could speak were able to recognise pictures. The representational function of language and pictures therefore arises at about the same time.

Another remarkable phenomenon that has attracted much attention is that many children as often as not look at their picture books upside down. Investigations have shown that pictures of people, trees, houses, ships, etc , which are turned through 90⁰ or 180⁰ are recognised

[1] Cf. the observations of E. Köhler in *Die Persönlichkeit des dreijährigen Kindes*, Leipzig, 1926.

as easily and as correctly as in the normal position. This agrees with the observation that beginners in drawing quite often make the same mistake about the orientation of objects in space, drawing people, or animals, or a cart with wheels, upside down. This also appears sometimes in the early spontaneous attempts of the child to write. More often, however, one finds in these another kind of inversion of orientation, mirror writing, in which left and right are interchanged. All this is a rather remarkable group of facts which goes to show that, within limits, the appreciation of spatial forms takes place independently of their orientation. Even when the child is able to draw the various forms, it often neglects their orientation. A more accurate theoretical and experimental investigation of these facts may possibly lead to valuable contributions to the theory of the perception of size, which has been discussed above, and the problem of the appreciation of form.

Psychologically, *rhythm* and *melody* in the field of time perception stand on the same level as spatial forms. We know that the effect of rhythmical sounds on a child of six months is different to that of a rhythmic sound. Rhythm is more strongly pleasurable and attracts the attention far more, and this interest grows during the first years.[1] Some children even react to rhythmical acoustic impressions with lively bodily movements, though it is only during the second year that the two begin to synchronize.[2] The process of perceiving, recognizing and repeating melodies starts, as a rule, still later. But here great individual differences make their appearance and one can usually judge quite early whether a child will be 'musical' or not. There seems to be trustworthy evidence about children who, at the age of two, could

[1] Cf. B. Löwenfeld, "Die Reaktionen des Säuglings auf Klänge und Geräusche," *Zeitschr. f. Psychol.* c (1926).

[2] With regard to the difficulty that the child has in imitating rhythmically and carrying out the spontaneous rhythmical movements it produces itself, cf. M. Guernsey, "Nachahmung in den ersten zwei Lebensjahren," *Zeitschr. f. Psychol.* cvii (1928).

correctly repeat simple melodies. On the whole, however, correct repetition of even the simplest and shortest melodies appears much later. It is probable that here, too, perception outdistances creation, for if we whistle to the two-year-old a song whose words are familiar to him, he is often able to recite some of the words, which proves that the melody and its rhythm have been recognized. Werner has written an exemplary and interesting paper on the development of melodic games and inventions of children between the ages of 2¾ and 5 years, but we cannot summarize his results within the limits of this chapter.[1] The language of the child ought to be recorded in the same way from its very first manifestations, in order to get hold of those aspects of rhythm and melody that appear so clearly in language and are of such importance to its expression. The common phrase ' the music (melody) of language ' is not quite applicable, in that neither adults nor children intentionally use definite intervals (second, third, fourth, etc.). When we speak of the melody of a sentence, we merely mean the rise and fall of the speaking voice, without regard to definite intervals. If I am not mistaken, this also holds for the child's first attempts at singing.

Examples of other types of forms (*Gestalten*) perceived very early by the child are various *forms of motion* and probably groups of touch sensations. The sense of touch probably gives rise to the first spatial figures. Blindfolded children are usually better able to recognise complicated bodies such as human faces by means of touch than unpractised adults. The reason for this is probably that in later years the sense of sight is over-emphasized, while the sense of touch and form in the hand makes relatively little progress.

(c) *Quantities, groups, series, numbers. What is the use of numbers?* When this question is asked in discussions

---

[1] H. Werner, "Die melodische Erfindung im frühen Kindesalter." *Abh. der Wiener Akad. d. Wiss. Philos. Hist. Kl.*, Vol. CLXXXII, 4 (1917).

on the theory of numbers, it refers to their function and tries to discover their nature. But here we are asking what they mean to the child and how the first steps into the realm of numbers are taken. If we understand both questions properly, we shall perhaps find that they are not very different. For centuries two principal methods have been advocated: the 'object lesson' (*Anschauungsmethode*) and the method of 'counting' (*Zählmethode*), and in traditional educational practice these two are even now the objects of heated controversy. It seems to me, however, that there is no real basis for this controversy; for a one-sided adherence to either method is justified neither by the natural development of the concepts of number (*Zahlfunktionen*) in the child, nor by the results of an analysis of mental arithmetic in adults. On the contrary, it is quite certain that there are at least two independent roots of the concept of number, the *conception of groups* and the *practice of arrangement in series*. Expressions such as pair, triplet, quadruplet, etc., exactly indicate what we mean by the name 'groups.' During its second to fourth year the child spontaneously learns to appreciate and distinguish pairs, triplets and later numerical units. This development probably does not go beyond the conception of a quadruplet. Simultaneously, but without recognizable relations to the group concepts, there arise the serial arrangements. But let us start at the beginning.

The first phenomenon to be noticed in this connection is that the child misses one of the constituents of a collection of things. Perhaps the *collection* (*Menge*) is a third concept in the mind of the child, next to that of a group and a series. An example may make this clear: a child in the beginning of its second year plays with three similar things, which it does not distinguish individually, e.g., three beans or coins. During a momentary diversion one of these is taken away. The child misses it, hunts for it and demands it back. A variation in the position of the three objects shows that it is not a gap in the visual image or a diminution in the area covered by them which is noticed by the child. It must be that the variety of possible manipulations—which may be identical with the idea of a collection—also finds expression in the optical impressions of the child, so that it is able to notice a diminution immediately, i.e., before taking up its game again. At any rate, one of the necessary conditions for the success of the experiment is that, what the child does with these objects, should depend on this variety of possible manipulations. A child, with whom this experiment had just been successfully carried out, was given three sweets, which were immediately taken from him again. He wept, but was afterwards perfectly satisfied on being given one of the sweets and allowed to eat it. He did not even ask for the others. In order, therefore, that the child's desire for eating should be satisfied, one thing was adequate, and during the eating of it the others were forgotten. Just as in the case of the cat mentioned on page 8, the number of possibilities which is mastered does not exceed three, but it soon grows rapidly. Preyer's report of a child (which was not investigated by himself) sounds rather improbable. He says : " One could not take away one of nine skittles without the child noticing this (its age being then ten months !) and when it was 1½ years old, the child knew at once whether one of its ten wooden animals was missing " (*Die Seele des Kindes*, p. 213). We cannot see from his statement what was at the bottom of this ' at once.' If, e.g., the animals all belonged to a Noah's ark, in which every one was different and had its appointed place, we could interpret this very simply as missing something which is not in its proper place, i.e., as a not especially remarkable achievement of memory (cf. p. 89).

We see, therefore, that premature interpretations can lead us thoroughly astray. This is also true of certain remarkable achievements of primitive peoples. It is said, for instance, that shepherds who cannot count very far will nevertheless miss one animal out of a very large flock. But it may be that the animal in question has some special characteristics, or that every animal in the flock is accustomed to some particular place. More remarkable are those games in which one man throws a handful of coins or beans on the ground, while his partner has at once to state their number. Here the chances for both players are more or less equal, so that the result cannot depend on pure guesswork or rapid counting. It must rest somehow on a certain sensitiveness to the number in a large collection and it is conceivable that an aptitude has here been trained to high perfection, which has atrophied in more civilized human beings. If I am not mistaken, the first step into the realm of numbers that is taken by animals and by the child, leads in this direction.

Towards the end of its second year, the child recognises the first group with a definite name, the *pair*. It begins to understand the duality of gloves, stockings, eyes, legs, and soon it is able to order such things in pairs. A little later it attains to a knowledge of groups of three and of numerical unity. The child does not advance beyond the concept of a trinity. When it appears to have grasped the four and five of domino blocks, it is configurations (*Gestalten*) and not real groups, which are concerned. Psychologically, it is true, configurations and groups are related ; but they are not exactly the same thing. A child can, and in fact does, grasp the three-cornered or four-cornered character of a figure, without actually realizing the triplet or quadruplet constituted by the sides or corners. The impressions of true configuration probably arise in the animal long before group impressions. I should hesitate, for instance, merely on the basis of the learning experiments, to attribute to the pecking fowl described on p. 8 a true conception of groups.

Finally, we come to the formation of *series*. The *one*, *two*, etc., which adults pronounce during rhythmical activities (e.g., when the child learns to walk) are very soon repeated by the child. The same thing happens when a number of objects is set up in a row and is also imitated by the child. One can often hear the little ones repeat in their spontaneous games, *one, two,* and then generally in any order, *seven, four, ten,* etc. The names by which numbers receive their specific functions of counting are given them not because of certain qualities, as is the case in names like *papa, mama, bow-wow,* but by the separate acts of setting up a series. At first they are probably not names for the objects arranged in series, but accompanying phenomena, expressions accompanying the act of ordering in a series. This enables us to understand three facts, which can be verified by anyone : first, that the similarity of the objects facilitates the repetition of words accompanying the series. The child is not distracted and sidetracked on to the familiar business of naming, because all the objects have the same name. Secondly, that which has already been done with coins, say, is easily applied to beans or anything else, whereas, thirdly, it is considerably more difficult for the child to apply the same accompanying words to another set of serial actions. A boy, who had learnt to say the numerals when showing the separate fingers of his own hand, on being asked to ' count ' the fingers of someone else, said : " I don't know that, I can only count my fingers " (age 4 ; 5). This is perfectly intelligible, because to do that, he would have had to perform a completely different series of movements.

How and when the correct order is introduced into the series of number-names, is a question as to the mechanism of association, which is of minor importance here. Much more important is a step forward taken by the child itself, which probably appears as a retrogression to most laymen. One will suddenly hear a monotonous *another one, another one, another one,* etc., *ad infinitum.* In this the similarity of the serial acts is expressed, and the child of its own accord recapitulates the most primitive stage in counting, which has only apparently been missed through the use of numerals. Now whether ' another one ' or numerals are used in setting up a series, there is one thing which takes a long time to develop : the ability to grasp the series as *a whole* " When five fingers are held up in front of her, and she is asked ' how many fingers are there ? ' she says : *I'll count them*, and counts correctly from one to five. If, as soon as the last number is spoken, she is asked, ' well, how many are there ? ' she begins to count afresh and so on a number of times " (age, 3 ; 7, from an observation by Stern). The child does not in the least understand what else beside ' counting ' is expected of it. This observation has been made again and again. Primitive peoples " often use different numerals for collections of things " (Wertheimer) belongs to the same category. In connection with this a further fact has to be noted : the establishment of series leads directly to ordinal numbers. When, at a certain period, one demands three of the objects which have been counted by the child, it gives you the *third* one, that is to say, the numerals have now become names that are given to the various objects according to their position in the series. Impressions of collections or of groups, on the other hand, are the preliminary steps in the acquisition of cardinal numbers. Ordinal and cardinal numbers, therefore, have different psychological roots and the child has subsequently to learn how to connect these two independent functions of words which signify numbers.

REFERENCES :

K. Bühler, *Die Gestaltwahrnehmungen*, Vol. I, 1913. W. Stern, " Über Verlagerte Raumformen," *Z.f. angew. Ps.* II. (1919). Decroly et Degrand, " Observations relatives à l'évolution des notions de quantités continues et discontinues chez l'enfant." *Arch. de Psychol.* xii (1912). H. Beckmann, " Die Entwicklung der Zahlleistung bei 2-6 jährigen Kindern, *Zeitschr. f. angew. Psych.*, xxii (1923).

CHAPTER FOUR

MEMORY AND IMAGINATION OF THE CHILD

PROBLEMS of the greatest theoretical importance are involved in the first appearance of concepts. Our concepts arise from our perceptions and are so similar to them, that Psychology can only distinguish differences of degree between these two modes of experience. Nevertheless, in the adult the two spheres, perceptions and conceptions, are on the whole quite separate. Indeed, they have to be separate if confusions that are dangerous to life are not to ensue. Hallucinations and illusions are not the rule in normal life. How do matters stand in the young child? For theoretical reasons we assume that it has to learn this distinction. The ' fibs ' of childhood are known to everyone. A little mite of three or four will tell us in all seriousness that he has met a bear on his walk, and the like. These things must not be regarded as serious moral lapses, for the child has a vivid imagination and often *cannot* distinguish memories from events which have been merely imagined. Similarly some writers assume—and probably correctly—that in very early childhood no hard and fast line can be drawn between immediate sense impressions and reproduced contents of consciousness, that is, between percepts and concepts.

In a girl one and a half years of age I have noticed a phenomenon which may be of this type. The child had returned from a walk and was toddling about on its own. Suddenly she remained rooted to the spot in the middle of the room. Her arms were bent at the elbows and held away from the body like the wings of a young bird, her eyes were wide open and staring. In a high, trembling voice, without the least modulation, and with obvious excitement, she uttered the words *daten lala*, which signify soldiers (*Soldaten*) and singing. She repeated this five or six times in exactly the same way, until I was able to distract her attention. No soldiers were to be heard singing, in the whole situation there was absolutely nothing that, as far as we could see, reminded her of soldiers or of singing. But three quarters of an hour before this, the child had been for a walk with the nurse and they had encountered some singing soldiers. Although she was quite familiar with this, it always gave her great pleasure. Nothing out of the ordinary had occurred. What, then, was happening to the child? The nervous excitement had been so intense, that with the utmost care we avoided anything which might stimulate her memory afresh. Nevertheless the whole scene was re-enacted that same evening. On the next two days, during which it rained, so that the child could not have heard any singing soldiers, it was repeated several times with gradually decreasing intensity. We can say at least one thing, that probably a very lively inner recurrence of the event had been taking place. Just as we sometimes cannot get rid of some important or even banal thought, e.g. a melody, which keeps on bothering us like a troublesome fly, so this event forced itself again and again into the consciousness of the child. Science has called this *perseveration*. The remarkable thing about it is the excitement, for which there was no apparent reason, as the child had many memories of a similar kind. Without systematically examining all the possible explanations, I should like to put forward the following formulation : it seems to me quite thinkable that, for the first time, the child noticed *how the lively inner recurrence of the event contrasted with the present perceptual situation*. The two did not correspond at all and it was this novelty which caused the excitement. During the next few weeks we noticed several similar occurrences, but without the whole nervous system being upset. If our interpretation is correct, we may see in such occurrences the travail and birth of the *conscious* distinction between perception and imagination. Further observations are urgently required.[1]

We cannot say for certain whether animals have an independent conceptual life. If we watch sleeping pointers 'dreaming', we might be inclined to assume that they are imagining themselves to be pursuing game. Horses are also said to dream. But in the psychological interpretation of such observations we must exercise great care. The majority of achievements brought about by training can be explained without assuming isolable images ; they are due to immediate association of definite sensory stimuli with definite bodily movements. Though we may be certain that memory is present when dogs dream, we are quite uncertain whether images are involved. At least we have no means of discovering whether there is in animals any conscious differentiation between immediate and reproduced sense impressions. Science, as Ebbinghaus has so truly remarked, must prefer the admission of honest poverty to the appearance of wealth. There are no reasons against attributing a developed imaginative life to the higher vertebrates, but there are also no decisive reasons for such an assumption.[2] The case of the human infant is very similar. What he can be trained to do does not allow us to formulate any definite theories. It is only when the child learns to speak and to understand what is spoken, that we can hope to gain more accurate information.

What the child produces when it relates something itself or listens intelligently to what is said, belongs to the

---

[1] For the theoretical questions involved, see : C. Stumpf, " Empfindung und Vorstellung," *Abhandl. d. Berliner Ak. d. Wiss.* 1918. J. Lindworsky, " Wahrnehmung und Vorstellung." *Z. Ps.* LXXX (1918) pp. 201 *et seq.*

[2] We must except the intelligent achievements of chimpanzees, which we cannot explain very well without conceptions. W. Köhler has collected several observations, which lead him to believe that chimpanzees have concepts like ourselves, but they are rare and at an extremely primitive stage of development.

chapter on *memory images*. From this time on, too, the child's play gives us an opportunity of watching the first products of *creative imagination*, which are greatly multiplied when it begins to enjoy hearing and reproducing short stories. *The period of fairy tales* is the most fruitful phase in the development of creative imagination in early childhood.

10.—THE MEMORIES OF THE CHILD

A memory contains more than the mere recalling of a previous experience. To have a real memory of something we must know that it has happened once before, under such and such outer and inner circumstances. To remember something perfectly, implies the correct reference of the object or situation to some particular point in our past. We think of a person, for instance, and know that we were at school with him, or that we met him at a certain time and place. Or a thought comes to our mind together with the knowledge of where we got it from and in what logical context it occurs. The latter implies a reference to the whole system of ideas that we have. This reference is not always as complete as we might wish it to be. We may, for instance, meet a man, and know that we have met him before and yet have not the slightest idea where, when or under what circumstances we met. This is called simple *recognition* by Psychology. A step lower than this is the *impression of being familiar with something*, which does not imply even the knowledge of whence this familiarity arises.

During its development, the young child passes through this series from the lowest to the highest. Impressions of familiarity and their correlate, impressions of strangeness, are experienced as early as the second month, and from then onwards, faces, rooms and other things, set up different reactions in the child.[1] In a strange room the

[1] Ch. Bühler, Hetzer, Mabel, " Die Wirksamkeit von Fremdheitsein drücken im ersten Lebensjahr," *Zeitschr. f. Psychol.*, cvii (1927).

infant opens its eyes wide and looks ' surprised,' while in its own nursery it behaves as though it is quite ' at home.' These reactions are, however, forgotten very quickly. If the mother goes away for even a fortnight, she becomes a stranger to the child.   When the child itself has been absent and returns to its room, it at first looks about wonderingly as though it were in the presence of something new, but before long everything is once more as it was. Attempts have been made to determine the ' span ' of familiarity and recognition and it has been found that in the first six months this only amounts to a few days, later to a few weeks and as early as the third year to several months.   Another not uninteresting problem is the duration through life of influences due to whole systems of impressions in early childhood.   When someone leaves his birthplace and home during his first year and returns to it as an adult, it can confidently be predicted that he will have no recollections of them.   But if he leaves during his second year, the matter is different.   Again, the man who at the same age comes into a different language environment, will later find his mother tongue totally strange to him.   But it is remarkable how quickly he begins to feel at home again phonetically.   He will learn to speak this language more rapidly and better than another foreigner, a proof that the early impressions have not been completely lost.

The first complete memories which have been described, those with spatial and temporal references, occur at the beginning of the second year and all of them bear a unitary character.   Some of them are supplements to the round of daily events in the life of the child.   Lunch, going for a walk, preparations for going to bed, all occur at definite times.   Now if one of the parts of these daily complexes happens to be omitted, if the mother, for instance, forgets to tie on the bib or allow the child to say ' good-night to father,' it will remind her of the omission.   What might be called the spatial completion of a well-known picture or situation is another aspect of this. A child regularly sees a dogcart on its walk. One day the cart is there without the dog. The child enquires about the dog and looks for him. Thirdly, memories of events which have only occurred once make their appearance. At first only fractions of an hour are involved. The child, for example, has been playing in the room with a ball which has rolled under a piece of furniture. It forgets about the ball and busies itself with other things. But after a while the child is asked about the ball, and at once runs to the spot where it ought to be. Or something exciting has happened, but the child has quieted down and no longer thinks about it. Soon after, the father comes home, the child remembers the whole affair again and relates it in his clumsy way.

The duration of a memory of such single events is largely dependent on the strength of the interest and the affects of the child that they originally called up. Uncle Doctor, for example, who puts a spoon into the child's mouth, usually leaves a fairly deep impress on its memory, so do celebrations in which it has taken an active part. But even during the second year it is rare for such events that only occur once, to leave behind memory traces for more than a few weeks. In the third year the duration may extend to several months, and in the fourth year there is no upper limit to the time for which special events are remembered. From what age exceptional impressions are likely to be remembered for the rest of one's life, is a question that has to be investigated in adults. *Enquêtes* have frequently been conducted on this problem and cases have been found where memories of special events reach back into the second year. What constitutes an exceptional impression will, naturally, have to be determined from the standpoint of the child. Often the important moments were ones of which no notice would be taken by adults. That is why, too, it is very difficult to obtain objective checks on the date of such events. It is easiest to obtain a check if a death or removal to another house occurred at the same time. It is worth noting that, during puberty, the adolescent actively busies himself with his own early childhood and brings to light much that seemed to have been forgotten. But this does not as yet lead to a connected and clear account of the years of childhood ; that is only produced during old age, when interest in the present begins to fade. Then the gaps are closed, the accounts of others and various historical sources serving to fill them. Where some gaps still remain, imagination completes the picture into one in which poetry and reality mingle.

REFERENCES :

CL. and W. STERN, *Erinnerung, Aussage und Lüge in der ersten Kindheit*, 1909. V. and C. HENRI, " Enquête sur les premiers souvenirs de l'enfance," *Année psychol.*, *vol.* III (1897). W. KAMMEL, " Über die erste Einzelerinnerung. Eine experimentelle Untersuchung," *Pädag. psychol. Forschungen*, 1913. H. REICHARDT, *Die Früherinnerungen als trügende kindliche Selbstbeobachtung in den ersten Lebensjahren*, Halle, 1926.

11.—THE IMAGINATION OF THE CHILD AT PLAY

When adults aimlessly give themselves up to the play of their imagination, day-dream, as we say, or when they are scheming, building castles in the air, they usually need complete rest or some purely automatic occupation. The gates of the senses must either be closed or must admit no impressions which could dominate the flow of images. The best travelling companions into the realm of phantasy for women used to be their knitting. In the small child the case is different. It needs impulses from outside, otherwise the threads soon break off and the mechanism of imagination comes to rest. *The child needs sense impressions and bodily activity to stimulate its spontaneous imaginative activity*, and finds both in play, as when it puts on a top hat, takes a stick in its hand and imitates the grown-ups. Such games are called *games of illusion*, because it is the illusion, which from a psychological point of view, is their most important factor. We are dealing here with the phenomenon of make-believe.

The child pretends to be grown-up. Like the actor it is playing a part, it pretends that the piece of wood is its darling baby which has to be carefully tended, or that the chair is a coach which is driven from the high box. In other words, it assigns a rôle to lifeless objects or to its animal pets and playmates and demands that this shall be carried out.

Let us take a glance back at earliest childhood and at the animal kingdom. Play and youth, with their preparation for the seriousness of life belong together, biologically. Organisms with plastic, uncompleted dispositions have to perfect themselves by practice. The very simplest and earliest games of the child are intended to develop its sense organs and its organs of motion. The child experiments with things, looks at them, feels them from all sides, smells them, and taps them to produce sounds. During a certain phase of its play it loves to take them to pieces and later even attempts to put them together again. In short, it behaves—somewhat unsystematically, it is true—like the scientist in his laboratory. Karl Groos has therefore aptly called these first games, *games of experiment.* Games of illusion stand at a slightly higher level, but we must not imagine that they represent something specifically human. When young puppies, kittens, or other predatory animals, chase and stalk each other as they would their prey, and then do not bite in earnest ; when a cat treats a ball like a mouse, to an external observer they also act 'as if.' These are first steps towards the make-believe of our children. Creative imagination can hardly be concerned in this even in the highest vertebrates, since their imaginative life is as yet far too primitive. So we see that the games of young predatory animals always take up definite forms, which only in the higher apes become more varied, and adjust themselves to the given circumstances. As we know from the dictionary of human epithets, the ape imitates his own kind, human beings, and other animals. W. Köhler has described a charming idyll to illustrate this, in his book on the chimpanzees. After the animals had learnt how to use a stick, this or anything which could be used as a stick, became their favourite toy. They poked about in every crack and hole and also at all insects that crawled about them. Now there were a lot of ants. In front of the bars of the cage ran a much used ant road. The chimpanzee poked at this with a straw. Some ants crawled up the straw, which the chimpanzee drew through its mouth. He liked the taste of acetic acid and so a regular game was developed : holding the straw until a sufficient number of ants had crawled up it, then drawing it through the mouth. Soon, on a sunny day when the ants were busy, the whole crowd of apes could be seen sitting next to each other, as intent on catching ants as the fisherman at a stream.

The illusionary games of the child are based on imitation to a far higher degree than are those of the chimpanzee. There is really only one game played by children that may be said to be defined and circumscribed by instinct ; it is playing at nursing or with dolls, chiefly practised by girls. Everything that happens in the family, and later on, everything the child hears about, is repeated in play. These ' dramatic games of imitation,' as they have been called, are of great value to the mental development of the child. For it is not only the outward manners of adults which the child acquires in this way. We may be sure that through this gate there enter into the soul of the child a large part of the affects and emotional responses, the attitude towards objects and the treatment of men and things, sympathies and antipathies. *For the child enters into the game with every fibre of its being.* Just as it projects its own feelings and emotions into other persons and things, so it enters into affects and feelings that it has at first only superficially imitated from adults, when they fit into the part the child is playing. Nevertheless, as every-day experience convinces us, the child very rarely confuses the reality of play with the reality of life, in spite of this active inner participation. *The sham interpretations of 'make-believe' are not false interpretations,* nor are they illusions in the pathological sense of the word. However firmly the child may insist that everyone else should join in keeping up the pretence of treating the piece of wood like a child, or of calling the chair a coach, the little player would nevertheless get a big shock if the doll she is trying to calm really began to cry, or if any toy really carried out its imaginary motions. When a hidden mechanism unexpectedly produces such movements, or, worse still, such sounds, the child draws back in panic. Often a simple deflection of its interest is sufficient to make the child itself treat the object with which it is playing as that which it really is. For instance it will throw into the fire a piece of wood, which a moment ago 'was' a beloved baby. Genuinely false interpretations would have entirely different consequences. K. Lange was the first to draw our attention to the fact that this is similar to the æsthetic illusions of adults during a play in the theatre, or while reading a book, or while absorbed in the contemplation of a work of art. In spite of deep absorption in its game, the child retains, at the back of its consciousness, the correct orientation towards the realities of life and even when it is in this absorbed state, it is able to tear the magic veil of illusion from things by a simple act of thought. When this is no longer possible, a pathological state of things is being approached.

Though we have many an excellent observation and sympathetic description of the games of children, the psychological analysis, especially of make-believe, is as yet full of shortcomings. For instance, we cannot say anything certain about the rôle of images in play. An event which the child is relating to us may sometimes be vividly present to his inner eye, but this succession of images can in no sense be compared to dreams. For in a dream everything that is imagined becomes reality. As I have already indicated, this is not the case in games. It is psychologically almost unthinkable what would happen if a world of images, seemingly real, were to surround and intermingle with the things objectively experienced. There would be no end to confusion. It is questionable whether there are more imaginative processes present in the child's mind when it is apparently manipulating objects that are not present at all—e.g., when it counts out coins in its shop or sings an invisible doll to sleep in its arms—than the shadowy and fleeting impressions experienced by adults in similar situations. If this state of things were comparable to a dream or to hypnosis, the child ought to be completely under the influence of its imagined situations, whereas in play it is their absolute master. In play, the child lets the train run over him or climbs into the lion's cage, but in a dream he would not do this in the same way at all. In short, I agree with W. Wundt in believing that the objectivity and vividness of imagination in play has been rather exaggerated. But let me emphasize that there are no conclusive arguments for or against this view.

Another undecided question is how the child comes to make-believe. I believe that we can partially understand this from a biological point of view. It is attributed to the continuation into conscious life of the sham games of animals. But this does not define, or at least does not completely make clear the psychological factors on which this type of behaviour is based. When a child looks at a picture book it also makes interpretations, such as ' that is a man,' ' that is a cow,' ' he is doing this.' But these are interpretations that are meant seriously. When the second period of ' asking why ' is entered, the child also wants explanations of things and events that are intended to be serious. Very often it invents its own, as in the following story about a three-year-old boy. Somehow he had stumbled on the problem of where all the dogs come from that run about the streets of Stuttgart. He said: "In the north of Berlin (the boy's wonderland) there are hares and dogs on the roof. They climb up with a ladder and play about with each other there . . . and then . . . and then a telephone appears, you know, a long rope, and on this they walk to Stuttgart. That is why they are with us." Groos, who tells this story, is quite right in comparing it with the simplest nature-myths of primitive peoples, like this Australian one : " Once upon a time," an Australian relates, " this pied bird was quite black. One day he had to go to war and began to paint himself white for the battle. But when he had only half finished, the enemy came, so that the bird had to go into the fight half black and half white. *That is why* all his descendants have these peculiar feathers." These are primitive attempts at explanation, which are at least meant seriously by their inventor. The little yarns with their apparent explanations that the child tells during play, are not even meant seriously by their originator. That is to say, they have not got the character of myths, but of *fairy tales*. It would be very valuable to know more accurately which one comes first in the child, or, to express it more cautiously, to know whether they are connected, and if so, how, because in race psychology a controversy is still going on as to whether fairy tales or nature myths are to be considered as earlier and more primitive, and in what way they are related.

REFERENCES :

K. Groos, *Die Spiele der Tiere*, 1896. *Die Spiele des Menschen*, 1899. *Der Lebenswert des Spiels*, 1910. *Das Seelenleben des Kindes*, ch. VII. H. Hetzer, " Das Volkstümliche Kinderspiel," *Wiener Arb. z. päd. Psy.* VI (1927). Idem, " Die symbolische Darstellung in der frühen Kindheit," *Wiener Arb. z. pädag. Psych.* III, 1926.

12.—FAIRY TALES AND THEIR RELATION TO THE CHILD'S FANTASIES

Our classical fairy tales have not been written by children nor for them ; nevertheless we seem to sense in them the soul of the child. The stories collected by the brothers Grimm throughout Germany, had been transmitted solely by grandmothers, mothers and nurses, through two, three or even more centuries. They were for the most part no longer literature for adults, but had taken their right to existence from a tradition kept up for the sake of children. It is not to be wondered at, therefore, that fairy tales had in many respects adapted themselves to the needs and standards of childish imagination. Here and there we can even follow this process of adaptation historically, as in the beautiful tale of the sleeping beauty (*Dornröschen*), which in its traditional German version has completely discarded its original erotic dress. But this by no means exhausts the possible explanations. Fairy tales are far more intimately related to the fantasies of the child and we can see this in all folk tales the world over. The central principle is no doubt that *fairy tales represent the first, or one of the first forms of artistic stories arising during the childhood of humanity.* In 1916 I made the suggestion in one of my lectures, that the child and its fairy tales should be examined under the magnifying glass of psychological analysis. This suggestion led to the work of my wife, on which the following is based.

(a). *The age of fairy tales.* The age of fairy tales of our children begins about the fourth year and lasts according to the type of education they receive. As a rule, Grimm's tales are outgrown by mentally well-trained and well stimulated children of educated town circles (who are sometimes pushed forward rather too rapidly) about the eighth or ninth year, to be replaced by more artificial ones like those of Andersen. Country children and others who are not pushed ahead so rapidly, keep their interest in the former kind up to their thirteenth or fourteenth year, according to some experienced teachers. Fairy tales are the most important, though not necessarily the very first, literature of childhood. Before that our youngest ones already evince interest in another type of story, which intelligent mothers invent themselves and others get out of good (or bad) children's books. There is a German book which has probably allowed for the needs of this period in the best way—*Struwwelpeter.* Its importance lies in the strong connection with personal

H

experiences of the child. The everyday happenings of the nursery are enumerated, and interspersed with those rules and warnings given to the child that has to learn to submit consciously to the demands of etiquette ruling civilized life. A little rhythm, rhyme, and grotesque humour are added as spices—although it is questionable whether much of this is appreciated. It is to be noted that the psychologically salient feature of Struwwelpeter-tales—the direct reference of the story to one's own person—leads into the beginnings of the fairy tale period. The first fairy tales have to be richly endowed with personal references : *a child, as small as you are,* etc. Later on this ceases to be necessary, because the child becomes able to turn its interest to the strange figures as such.

A further step in development terminates the fairy tale period. During the ' hobbledehoy age,' as we all know, stories of pirates and Red Indians begin to interest our children, particularly boys. A better example of this kind of literature is the classic, *Robinson Crusoe.* What distinguishes this from fairy tales ? Of the many points of distinction the following are probably the most important : *Robinson Crusoe is close to actuality,* it is realistic. With almost scientific accuracy and care the inventions are described, by means of which the man that has only himself to rely upon masters wild nature, whereas the fairy tale is *strange to reality,* idealistic, takes place anywhere and at any time, without in the least bothering whether the related events are true to the laws of nature or of mental life. A fairy tale above all is imaginative art, whilst in Robinson Crusoe, critical thought plays an important part. That is why the real enjoyment of a fairy tale demands a specific attitude, which the child finds impossible later when it has lost its naïve ways of thinking. It is only the adult who regains the correct relationship to fairy tales.

(*b*). *Psychological analysis.* Let us proceed to the analysis of these curious stories. If we wish to use them for obtaining an insight into the mental life of the child, we must first of all learn to classify their contents from a psychological standpoint, that is, we must understand *what* is related, and *how* it is set out. I shall only indicate the main headings. The *number of characters* in Grimm's fairy tales is small and very homogeneous. The chief actors are children, and young persons of a marriageable age, who are nevertheless still regarded as children. Father, mother, grandmother, the royal pair, and workmen form a kind of background. The *stepmother* is more important, often approaching in interest the witches. Most important are *fabulous beings*, dwarfs, giants, and witches. All the personages are drawn as *types having only one or two outstanding characteristics*, like great bodily size or smallness, strength or weakness, beauty or ugliness, together with those moral characters which are praised or censured in a young child : good and evil, obedience and disobedience, industry and sloth, modesty, stupidity and a few more. Dullness or simplicity do not necessarily always appear in an unfavourable light, but are often drawn very sympathetically and triumph in the end. The characters are differentiated from one another by *simple contrast* in character or fate. Luck and misfortune are distributed according to the clear and intelligible rule that virtue must triumph in the end and vice be punished. The *animals* in the fairy tale (not in animal fables) are superior to man in some respects and enter on the scene as helpers and saviours, avengers and judges, somewhat like the fabulous beings. In the tale it is on these that the special interest of storyteller and listener is concentrated. They usually appear at some unexpected moment, bringing help or disaster. At any rate they always are a deciding factor, and sometimes guide the threads of events from the outset.

The ' *milieu* ' of fairy tales is the world of imagination of the youngsters, which they know from their own experience ; the magnificent court of the king, of which they form a picture from hearsay ; the dark forest and imaginary places in which these legendary beings move. Poverty and wealth are in sharpest contrast, nevertheless the characters pass from one to the other without the slightest difficulty. The beggar maid who becomes a queen, immediately knows how to behave herself in accordance with her new station, and the princess has to go begging. But a fairy tale does not pay too much attention to the environment ; the whole interest is concentrated on the action.

The *action* (except in humorous or animal stories) centres around *miraculous events*, transformations, rescues, the solution of almost insoluble tasks by means of unheard of bodily and mental powers. All of these are, psychologically speaking, of a *sensational* kind, something absolutely different to every-day life and so satisfying the imagination of primitive man, which is continually seeking after something new. A miraculous happening is the turning point of the story. The *motives* for the actions spring from the simple and primitive will. Most of the events are born out of the affect of the moment, and that is why fairy tales are so full of caprice. Where a person intrudes, for example, he is removed, whether he is guilty or not. Everything happens quickly, reward and punishment follow immediately on the deed and generally consist in something tangible, a beautiful bride, the crown, or corporal punishment, poverty, and death. Where the action does not take place immediately after some affect, it occurs as the result of some order. The moral code is based on a healthy, sometimes rough but never weakly conception of *authority*.

The *technique* of telling a fairy tale consists in splitting up the action into almost independent single events, strung together like pearls and made coherent by methods of style that are continually repeated. The most popular use of this method is to place some disposition at the beginning, in the form of a prophecy or an order commanding or forbidding something to be done, that, after it has been given, is bound to be transgressed. Once this has been laid down as the structural plan, the rest can consist of separate pictures going by—somewhat like a modern film—that do not need to be interrupted by explanations. Another much used method is repetition in different forms. In the so-called 'double fairy tales' for instance, there are two sets of actors and the second set always experiences and attains exactly the opposite to the first. Or it may be that difficult tasks are only completed at the third attempt, or by three different heroes. In these repetitions we see quite clearly how everything has to proceed according to the original disposition, exactly as can be foreseen.

(c). *Conclusions.* A child listens to a good fairy tale with breathless interest. There is no doubt that in imagination it is present on the scene of action, relives the emotions of the heroes, hopes and fears with them, loves or hates them. The rather difficult psychological analysis of the life of emotions and the will in fairy tales has not as yet been attempted. But the following theorem, which cannot rest on mere chance, may be enunciated about the thought activity of the audience : *Certain achievements of the imagination are definitely encouraged by the fairy tale, which is adapted to them as to no other type of literature ; others are called into play by it only very slightly ; a third group is almost completely ignored.* Let us examine these three groups in more detail.

The fairy tale encourages *rapid and varied changes of the image content*, and it is full of sudden transformations of all kinds. The prince with the 'wishable thoughts' says to the bad cook : "'You shall become a black poodle, with a gold chain round your neck ; and you shall eat glowing coals, till the flames leap from your throat.' And when he had spoken these words, the old man was changed to a poodle, and had a gold chain round his neck, and the cooks had to fetch live coals for him to eat, so that the flames leapt from his throat.''

The prince has changed his bride to a carnation and is carrying her in his pocket at his father's table : " And he put his hand in his pocket and took out the carnation, and placed her on the table before the king. And she was more beautiful than any the king had ever seen. Thereupon his son said : ' now you shall also see her in her true form,' and wished her to be a maiden. There she stood and was so beautiful, that no artist could have painted her better."

Such little sorceries are repeated under many forms. The sudden translation to another place, the sudden appearance of new characters in the situation (*deus ex machina*), the transformation of the whole situation (*the magic table cloth*) all belong to this category. It is often like a dream. The imagination of the adult can easily follow all this, since it is not necessary that one idea should have faded before another has taken its place. The child enjoys such quick changes, but it must be remembered that this type of fairy tale (transformation stories) are not those preferred and demanded by the youngest children. The pleasure of quick changes in the image content has first to be acquired and practised. In fact, we may suppose that the utility, in a sense the biological purpose of such play, is that the stock of images should be made labile and easily controlled.

As against this, the fairy tale makes extraordinarily few demands on the power of *simultaneous combinations of ideas*, that is, the ability of being able to see the connection between two ideas presented at the same time. The fairy tale has to take into consideration the fact that the child's power of combination is very small. A large number of facts illustrate this : first, the many complex beings that the imagination of different peoples has evolved, like the sphinx, a maiden with the body of a beast of prey, the centaur, part man and part horse, the mermaid, part fish and part woman. None of these appear in German fairy tales for children. Even the devil, to whom popular imagination attributes horns, tail and a horse-hoof, comes on the scene in a mannerly way as a human being, for instance as a huntsman in a green coat. Angels with wings appear now and then, but I do not regard this as an exception, for the child can see wooden or stone effigies of such beings everywhere in the village and so does not need to conceive of them himself, which is what we are concerned with at the moment. Secondly, there is certainly no lack of descriptions of wealth and splendour in the palace of the king or in the land of the dwarfs. But if we look into this more carefully, we find that there is a succession in the imagery. It is never necessary to conceive of more than three or four things, animals, or persons, or attributes of things at the same time. Thirdly, the fairy tale is remarkably sparing in its transference of simple attributes from one thing to another. It is surprising, for instance, how seldom the natural colours of things are mentioned in Grimm's fairy tales. Tales such as Little Red Riding-Hood, in which a child is named after its red cap, or the wolf who is recognized by his black paws, which are then whitened with flour, are rare. On the other hand the world of fairy tales gleams and glitters out of dark caves and forests and the black night. *One* optical quality is poured over everything : there is nothing in the world which at one time or another does not become *golden*, plants, fruit, living animals, raiment, articles of common use, hair and other parts of the body, as well as everything else. It is improbable that the imagination can and should follow all this. Indeed, it would be possible to prove that a fairy tale occasionally expects that this does not happen. As long as something begins to shine at the right time, everything else can and does remain in its natural colours (which accompany the setting but are unnoticed).

Something else which flourishes in fairy tales and is used again and again, is the *method of exaggeration*. Every work of art accentuates and exaggerates, but in fairy tales this is carried to extremes. Its characters are angels of beauty and goodness, or utterly detestable ;

they live among untold riches or in abject poverty, have heaven or hell on earth and so on.   In this a certain intellectual primitiveness finds its expression, since crass contrasts are necessary for enabling the childish audience to distinguish the characters from one another and to take up a definite attitude of love or hate, approval or disapproval towards them.   It also expresses an æsthetic primitiveness, for the unexperienced being does not know where to stop in dwelling on anything which promises pleasure.   But the important point, as far as I can see, is that the child enjoys the process of exaggeration itself. This is evident from the constant *repetitions*, e.g., of the extraordinary smallness of the dwarf, and everything in his house, more so from the ' *going-one-better* ' and finally from the direct presentation of series, *scales* up and down which the imagination can run.   The pretty story is well known about ' The Fisherman and his Wife' (" For my wife, dame Isabel, wishes what I scarce dare tell "). They ascend from the miserable hovel in five stages to the palace of the pope.   At the emperor's throne " there stood his paladins, in two rows, one always smaller than the next, from the mightiest giant two miles high to the smallest dwarf, who was no larger than my little finger." The pope wears three crowns.   He sits on a throne, two miles high, and at his side there stand two rows of lights, " the largest as thick and as high as the biggest tower, down to the tiniest rush-light."   The child derives much pleasure from running up and down such scales.   It may be that it has to learn and practise such changes in size of its images during the ' fairy tale age.'

The fairy tale avoids *all thinking which is at all compli-cated.*   Any deeper connections are at most merely indi-cated and are probably perceived in some intuitive fashion by the child.   This is the field in which the hardest task falls to the school.   One of the intelligence tests for schoolchildren consists in comparing, for instance, a fly and a butterfly, or ice and wood.   Such simple tasks are found to offer unexpected difficulties to less advanced children. The perceptual comparisons which a child draws for itself are different. A boy, eight years of age, observes the motion of the long antennæ of a butterfly and explains that the animal is ' knitting socks ' (motion of knitting needles). This is no bad analogy, but also no great effort from a psychological point of view, merely an association by similarity. But if we ask what the difference is between ice and wood, the child has to find the points of similarity itself and bring the two things together in its imagination, which is no mean effort of abstraction. That is why poetic allusions, metaphors, etc. are completely absent in fairy tales. Only the simplest colloquial expressions are used, red as blood, white as snow, zig-zag like lightning, fast as the wind, slow like the snail, etc. Or descriptions like the following : Bearskin had not washed for several years and now " his hair covered all his face, his beard appeared like a piece of dirty cloth, his nails were claws, and his countenance was so covered with dirt that one might have grown cresses upon it."

REFERENCES :

F. v. d. LEYEN, *Das Märchen.* No. 97 in the series *Wissenschaft und Bildung,* 2nd edn. 1917. CHARLOTTE BÜHLER, " Das Märchen und die Phantasie des Kindes." *Beiheft* 17, *Zeitschr. f. angew. Psychol.* 1918, *2nd edn.* 1927. A. RUMPF, *Kind u. Buch,* 2nd edn., Berlin and Bonn, 1928.

CHAPTER FIVE

THE DEVELOPMENT OF DRAWING

WE owe some valuable information about the mental life of the child to the scribblings and drawings it begins to produce from about its fourth or fifth year. In 1887 the Italian art-historian C. Ricci, wrote an interesting and witty book about the drawings of children, which started assiduous investigations in this field. German art teachers, such as Konrad Lange, A. Lichtmark, and G. Hirth and H. Cornelius in Munich, have taken up and developed Ricci's ideas. Contributions have been made by Americans and Frenchmen, so that there is to-day a large literature on the subject of children's drawings. Extensive collections were made, among others, by the historian Lamprecht, in Leipzig. In 1895, J. Sully wrote a sound psychological survey in his book, "Studies of Childhood," which is still worth reading to-day. 1905 brought two large illustrated works, one by S. Levinstein, who belongs to Lamprecht's school, the other by the well-known Munich pedagogue, G. Kerschensteiner. Since then literary activity has cooled down somewhat. We need only mention two larger books, that of the Frenchman, G. H. Luquet (1913), and a very fine study by W. Krötzsch (1917), which filled in many gaps.

How should the drawings of children be studied? That depends on the particular end in view. At first, when it was necessary to obtain a general survey, the *art historian's method* sufficed. A collection of material, as comprehensive as possible was made ; the items being dated with certainty and the authors and their environment known. From this the general characteristics of the child's drawings were read off. The psychologist was more at home in the *biographical method*, which keeps to one child and tries to follow its whole development. The Americans, finally, with their tendency towards mass-production, have instituted extensive *enquêtes*. Whole classes were given definite tasks, and the results analysed by *statistical methods*. Nowadays, when our main concern is to make the psychological analysis of the act of drawing finer, we have to take the trouble to observe as accurately as possible the origin of every single drawing and all that accompanies it, as Krötzsch has recently done.

REFERENCES :

KONRAD LANGE, *Die Künstlerische Erziehung der Deutschen Jugend*, 1895. J. SULLY, *Studies of Childhood*, Ch. X., 1895. S. LEVINSTEIN, *Kinderzeichnungen bis zum 14. Lebensjahr. Mit Parallelen aus der Urgeschichte, Kulturgeschichte und Völkerkunde*, 1905. G. KERSCHENSTEINER, *Die Entwicklung der Zeichnerischen Begabung*, 1905. G. H. LUQUET, *Les dessins d'un enfant*, Paris, 1913. W. KRÖTZSCH, *Rhythmus und Form in der freien Kinderzeichnung*, 1917.

13.—PRELIMINARY STAGES

(*a*). *Scribbling*. In the first attempts at drawing, unlike in those of speech, there does not seem to be any collaboration with instincts. It is the instinct of imitation from which the first impulses come. The child sees its older comrades or adults drawing and writing and tries to imitate them. That is why the time at which drawing begins is so indeterminate and subject to large individual variations. It has been found to occur as early as the second year, in other cases as late as the fourth. At first these playful efforts are no more than an aimless gesticulation with some long object, be it spoon or pencil, but later, when the connection between the motions of the hand and the results on paper has been grasped, the child begins to derive pleasure from producing lines. The period of *scribbling* has begun. Because of its lack of meaning, this scribbling corresponds to the first ' cooings ' of the child.

(b). *Transition to representational drawings.* One day the child discovers in its criss-cross lines some shape, which reminds it of a familiar object, and so the second phase in the development of drawing begins. Scribbling now takes up a different meaning, we might call it the *real meaning*, that of drawing. The child wants to make pictures. On the whole this advance is psychologically similar to that from meaningless babbling to names, for in both, bodily movements that are practised in play receive a *representational function.* Once this step has been taken, a general result becomes apparent, if not after the first attempt, at any rate after two or three attempts. The effect is similar to that observed in adults who have reached some generalized conclusion. That is to say, the child makes its further efforts with the intention of portraying something. This is objectively apparent in the names that the child now begins to give to its drawings. They are no longer fortuitous ; different names are given to different figures and gradually become fixed. Moreover a drawing begins to show definite form. The child, for example, wishes to draw a man and explains that a certain arrangement of lines represents the head, others represent this or that. The representational intention is apparent in this differentiation long before there is any similarity in the picture to the object portrayed.

(c). *Scribble-ornamentation.* The simplest form of ornamentational design, called, ' scribble-ornament,' arises in primitive races out of this scribbling in play. Only a small step is needed for this transition. As soon as the interest and pleasure of playing is transferred from the mere activity of making strokes to its results, these lines must assume certain characteristics in order to stimulate interest and pleasure and keep them alive. We shall have a design before us, when these characteristics either belong to the lines themselves, or to something which fills up a space or completes neighbouring representational objects. This is more or less the case in childish drawing, except that the ornamentation which is discovered through the random drawing of lines, comes demonstrably later than representational drawing. In the very earliest drawings of children we look in vain for actual, original ornamentation, but later, at about school-going age, a strong desire for it develops and runs riot in the graphic productions of children.

REFERENCES:

MAJOR, *First Steps in Mental Growth*, Ch. III. LUKENS, " A Study of Children's Drawings in the Early Years." *Pedag. Sem.* IV (1896). SHINN, " Studies of Children's Drawings," *Univ. of California Studies in Psych.* II (1897). W. KRÖTZSCH, p. 102. A youthful talent for ornamentation is described by G. FR. MUTH, " Über Ornamentierungs-versuche mit Kindern im Alter von 6-9 Jahren," *Zeitschr. f. angew. Psych.*, 1912.

14.—THE SCHEMA

(a). *Objects and Style.* For a long time man and a few animals take preference among the objects depicted by the child. Only later do houses, carts, locomotives, etc., appear and often very late trees, flowers and articles of common use. Why does the budding artist attempt the most difficult things first ? The child does not as yet know any difficulties or the limits of its own capacity. The chief reason why it draws inspiration from human beings and animals must in some way be connected with the fact that they are alive and active. The child's well-being depends on them and it has to enter into relations with them. The same predilections are shown by primitive races. " The living, moving animal, attracts their attention to a far greater extent, and is more easily apprehended as a whole, than the plant, which consists of many leaves and flowers." (R. Andree, " *Das Zeichnen bei Naturvölkern.*").

The first human figures are sketchy and incomplete, unorganized and without proportions. An examination of Fig. 7, will be more instructive than laborious descriptions. At any rate, at this stage one can recognize outlines and above all a closed line for the head as well as the most important features. Out of the circle of the head other lines begin to grow, most frequently two straight

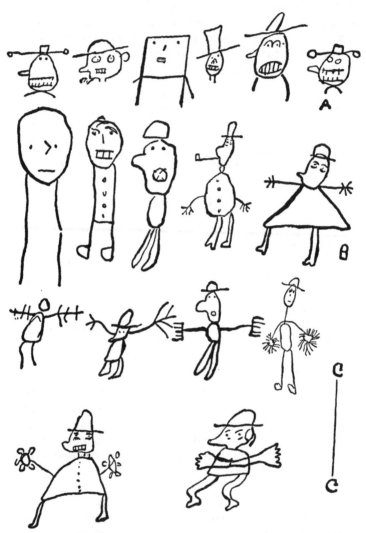

FIG. 7.—SCHEMATIC DRAWINGS OF CHILDREN. MAN. A: HEADS
B: BODIES AND LEGS; C: ARMS AND HANDS.
(Selected from *Sully*. Somewhat reduced.)

lines downwards, which are obviously meant to represent the legs. The arms are frequently missing, or come out of the head next to the legs. The torso and the neck are very badly treated. Later, the torso becomes merely a useful place " on which a head can be placed and from which limbs can be suspended." " This sounds absurd, since the arms belong to the body ; but for a child, the body merely plays the part of a hook on which everything can be hung" (Levinstein, p. 10). The first drawings of human beings are, without exception, full-face portraits. Later the profile becomes more and more important, and in a very characteristic fashion. One after another the various parts of the body are turned sideways, so that curious mixtures of full-face and profile portraits are produced. At the age of eight, according to Levinstein, about half of the primary school children draw such mixed figures, while later the profile view prevails almost completely.

Of the animal kingdom the young child usually draws only the familiar companions of man, dog, horse, cat, pig, cow. Sometimes it draws ' a large bird ' (goose, duck, fowl), or ' a small bird ' (pigeon, sparrow, swallow), and sometimes ' fishes.' Occasionally a gradual differentiation from some basic animal form or even from the human form has been observed, but such cases are not the rule. The animal is drawn from the very beginning in profile, head and body often in closed outline, legs and tail stuck to them. After a period in which mammals are given an unlimited number of legs, the correct number are drawn before the correct number of fingers are known ; this is obviously connected with the arrangement in two pairs, as three legs are seen very rarely.

Of the vegetable kingdom the tree takes first place. Its figure is originally like that of human beings and its development from a mere scrawl can be followed. It develops either in an anatomical way, that is, a gradual differentiation into trunk, branches with more and more twigs, leaves and fruit takes place, or the outline becomes gradually more tree-like, as this is easier to draw. The numerous different attempts of the child show us how difficult a simple matter like the shape of a fork in a branch can be for the child. Later on, when the child begins its designing and draws flowers, creepers and other leafy plants, the same problem of forked branches presents itself. Now and then it is found that children have only one pattern—like a stencil—for both trees and flowers.

Psychologically there is nothing new to be seen in the primitive outlines of *houses*. As is to be expected, the first to be represented is the front view, as a rectangle containing many windows and doors in any arrangement, with a triangular roof and numerous chimneys. The desire to depict more sides, arises very early and when the child has satisfactorily drawn three or four next to each other, it gets into difficulties over the roof.

In conclusion, let me say a few words about the composition of pictures. Two persons meeting each other and holding out their hands are placed independently, next to each other, as is fitting. Indeed, their independence is usually such that it becomes necessary to indicate, subsequently, how they belong together. But this does not worry the child in the least. It lengthens the arms until they meet, or simply draws a line joining the hands. Since the child has not yet realized the action of the joints, the whole arm, which is reaching for something, is bent as is the whole person that is supposed to be sitting down. The man on horseback is interesting. The main axes of the picture ($\perp$) are always drawn correctly but no more. We can see how the child is puzzled by the connection between the two figures. Sometimes the man is too high above the horse, sometimes he is half inside it ; and when the contour of the man's body is correctly rounded off by the back of the horse, the difficult problem of the legs begins, which is often solved in peculiar ways (cf. Fig. 8). The same difficulties are apparent in the pictures of a man in a boat or cart.

(b). *Analysis of the act of drawing.* Why does the child draw such curious outlines of things? Surely it sees them differently, or, more correctly, its retinal images are quite different. The obvious answer, " because they are easiest to draw and are drawn by the adult like

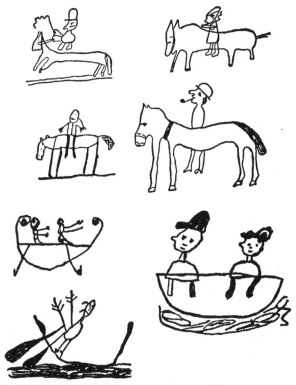

FIG. 8.—THE MAN ON HORSEBACK AND THE MAN IN A BOAT.
(Selected from *Sully* and *Ricci*. Somewhat reduced.)

that for the child to copy," contains some truth, but is not adequate. No doubt the clumsiness of the child's hands plays a part, as well as imitation. But even children who have practically no outside help, and all primitive peoples, with very few remarkable exceptions, draw in outline. There can be no doubt that, from the

I

point of view of the art of drawing, this childish schematism is an abortion, which runs counter to the spirit of pictorial art in many respects. If we once fall into this habit, it is very difficult to break ourselves of it. Indeed, we know that it is the bane of drawing masters, to get the child to *see* properly. They are quite right in saying that the child has been badly brought up, that it is in a rut out of which they can only drag it with the greatest difficulty. But it is no use complaining, and it would be a serious error to suppose that a radical change can be brought about by the ' back to nature ' method. Negro and Red Indian children can hardly be said to have lost contact with nature, yet they draw in just the same schematic way as our own children.

The root of the evil reaches far deeper into man's intellectual development. It is the fault of our *mastery of language*, which models the mind of man according to its requirements, and—do not let us be unjust !—enables us by virtue of that mastery to rise to the highest achievements of thought. As soon as objects have received their names, the formation of concepts begins, *and these take the place of concrete images.* Conceptual knowledge, which is formulated in language, dominates the memory of the child. What happens when we try to impress some event on our own memories ? As a rule the concrete images fade, but as far as the facts are capable of being expressed in language, we remember them. This development begins as early as the second year in the child and when it begins to draw—in its third or fourth year—its memory is by no means a storehouse of separate pictures, but an encyclopædia of knowledge. *The child draws from its knowledge, that is how its schematic drawings come about.* Here, then, we have the key to the understanding of children's drawings. Let us examine this in detail.

First : The child draws almost entirely *from memory,* ' out of its head ' as we say. If it wants to draw a man, it does not look around for a model or a copy, but cheerfully goes ahead with its task and puts into the drawing whatever it knows about a man and whatever comes to its mind. The man must have two eyes, even in profile, the horseman two legs. Clothes are hung round him afterwards, as one would clothe a doll. One can see what is in his pockets and the coins in his purse, as in an X-ray photograph. Models and copies at most serve as suggestive impulses. Let a child stand in front of a class, facing towards the right, and ask the class to draw it. You will be surprised how many children will draw a portrait facing left.

Secondly: The portrayed objects only receive *their constant and essential attributes* and these only in the forms which occur most often and are therefore *the dominant ones*. What is an arm? Its most important property, from the child's point of view, is that it can be stretched out sideways and can hold something. So the child draws a line from the body. It does not matter to what point this is attached. (Popular thought expresses this in words such as *Wandarm, Armleuchter, Hebelarm*). What is the mouth? The most elementary fact about it is that it is a slit or hole in the head. Therefore the child draws a circle, a rectangle or merely a line, within the circle representing the head. The most important and most familiar aspect of the hand is the front view, which allows most of its structure to be seen. Therefore, the child always draws a hand from the front and wrestles with the problem of how the fingers are attached to it. This method is carried to such lengths, that parts of the same thing appear next to each other in the picture in a way in which they would never be seen together. For instance the wheels of a cart may be drawn as circles and the body as a rectangle, as though seen from above, the table as a square with the legs at the four corners, pointing downwards. If a child is given a cube as model, it will rarely succed in drawing anything but squares that are joined to each other in some way.

Thirdly: We all know what the first essay of a child is like. Subject, " the horse ": "A horse has a head and a

tail. It has two legs in front and also two behind."
Now the order of a story is not necessarily the spatial
order of the objects it describes. If we read in a fairy
tale : " the dwarf had a huge head and two short little
legs, snow white hands and a nose like a glowing coal,"
we should certainly not criticize the style because of the
irregular order adopted. If such a sentence were to
guide the efforts of a child that does not see the picture in
its mind as a whole, we might expect that the short legs
will be drawn as growing straight from the head and the
hands likewise. The nose, again, might be put in its
proper place in the middle of the face. But that is
exactly what we see in some of the earliest pictorial efforts
of the child. Its drawings are, in a sense, *graphic accounts.*
Looked at in this way, the irregular order found in its
drawings becomes intelligible. We cannot simply assume
that the mind of the child is in a state of chaos, because if
these graphic accounts be translated into language, they
might be found to be well ordered. The fault lies not so
much in a chaotic mind, as in *errors of translating from
knowledge—formulated in language—to the spatial order of
pictorial representation.*

Fourthly : The child adds part after part, it draws
synthetically, as it remembers one thing after another.
Many of its impossible creations can be understood if we
remember this. They are errors of composition. Imagine
the principal parts of several human figures cut out of
different books and mixed together. If these parts are
now combined again, we shall obtain a chaos of proportions.
If we remember that something similar is happening in a
child's additive drawings, we shall better be able to
judge them. We find disproportions in size in them
everywhere, the most obvious one being that between the
head and the body of a human figure. The head is always
drawn too large. It may be that the exaggeration is
due to the child's special interest in faces, or the child
may draw a picture of the head from near by, since he has
had many opportunities of observing it at close quarters.

Nothing is known about this as yet. The other bodily proportions are also well worth investigating more accurately. It is remarkable that, as a rule, we find good symmetry, in spite of the mistakes in proportions. But that can easily be explained from the fact that the idea of symmetry is not derived from optical impressions, but from knowledge. The child knows that there are two equal eyes, ears, arms and legs, and accordingly draws them so. In this way the schema is developed.

REFERENCES:

The most complete collections of material are to be found in Levinstein and Kerschensteiner. For the psychological analysis, cf. Ricci and Sully, as well as Bühler, *Die geistige Entwicklung des Kindes*, 1918, 5th edn., 1929.

15.—THE REALISTIC PICTURE

(a). *The lines of development.* Starting from the mere outline, the 'schema,' four directions of development are theoretically possible. The first, as the history of mankind shows, leads to the *invention of writing*. In everyday use, the schema is filed down, simplified and made easy to write. It is subjected to the laws governing the evolution of tradition (i.e., the handing on from one generation to the next), so that it loses its original similarity to the object portrayed and approximates to a pure *symbol*. When these symbols begin to serve the practical purpose of imparting news, writing begins. Thus, to simplify his dealings with the white man, the Red Indian of North America invented a primitive kind of picture-writing, but it has fallen behind in comparison with the advancing civilization of the white man. I am not acquainted with Chinese writing, but the idea of the schema enables us to understand perfectly, how a single stroke in the compound symbols of this writing, can stand for an abstract concept, as I am told it does. It is supposed that first *sentence-writing*, then *word-writing* and finally, *writing by means of letters* were developed. Man must therefore at one time have made the fundamental discovery that not only things, but language as well, can be ' painted.' But it is readily understandable from a psychological point of view that in doing so, he first hit upon the most clumsy graphical method, whereby each sign has to represent a large number of facts, and only last on the brilliant method of syllable and letter-writing. The latter method has probably been discovered several times over in the history of mankind.[1]

The second line of development leads into æsthetics. Playing about with the various forms of the schema and selecting the most pleasing ones, produces a special type of ornamental design, which could be called the *typically schematic design*. In the case of the South American Indians we can clearly see how drawings of the human figure gradually lose their similarity to nature and their representational value, becoming mere ornaments. If one knows the schema, one understands without further explanation why this type of ornamentation should be subject to the principle of symmetry. There is no reason why the scribble-ornament, for example, should be symmetrical, but there is every reason why it, as well as other types of ornamentation, should occur with numerous repetitions.

The third line of development leads to ' working drawings ' in plan and elevation, and to the type of drawing represented by geographical maps. The schema, after all, is already a plan and its figures are plane. In the schema of the child, too, purely symbolic signs are used for certain details, a method which is systematically perfected in geographical maps. The common fundamental property of technical drawings and maps is topographical exactness, so that all the relations of size and direction can be measured directly with ruler and protractor. How this type of drawing has been developed in the course of racial evolution, I do not know. But among our own children, some have a precocious, one-sided talent for technical

<hr>

[1] Cf. Th. W. Danzel, *Die Anfänge der Schrift*, 1912 ; K. Weule, *Vom Kerbstock zum Alphabet* (" Kosmos " series) 1915.

drawing. Levinstein discovered a thirteen year old boy, who had been drawing locomotives passionately, with unceasing industry and great success ever since his fourth year. Another boy, only 6½ years of age, drew the steam engine plant of a bakery from memory, motor cars from all sides, electric trams and trains in almost pure elevation. He used a ruler for the straight lines, and at first drew circles by means of buttons, of which he had made a large collection in all sizes. No one had shown the child how to make technical drawings, he had hit on them himself. Though such achievements are remarkable, they do not present special psychological problems.

The fourth line leads, finally, to the realistic picture. ' Realistic ' I call a photograph, and with it every picture which is constructed *according to the principles of photography*, that is, above all with due regard for the perspective of form and size. Whether the portrayed object actually exists or not, whether the artist draws it from life or from memory, whether it has been reproduced as the artist saw it or has been transformed by his imagination, all this is irrelevant to the concept ' realistic.'

(b). *The actual course of development.* In the drawings of the average child we find indications of all this, but no more. As a rule, the desire for graphic expression *fades at the level of the schema*, unless there be special talent or school training. About the age at which the child outgrows fairy tales, it also gives up its spontaneous efforts at drawing. We can say that it discards schematic drawing just as it discards many other things of which later it almost seems to be ashamed, without being able to put something more mature in their place. The spontaneous beginnings of the art of drawing therefore atrophy quite soon, so completely, indeed, that if they were asked to draw a man or a horse, most members of the civilized nations of to-day would produce drawings hardly distinguishable from those of a child eight or ten years of age. These people have not tried to draw since their childhood. Their whole graphic ability lies in writing, and since this belongs to language, we may say : *Language has first spoilt drawing, and then swallowed it up completely.*

The old methods of teaching drawing, which I by no means wish to defend, cannot be made wholly responsible for this state of affairs, and the more recent methods, whose good results are certainly to be commended, must beware of illusions. There are differences of natural talent in all fields of mental achievement, but nowhere are they as striking as in music and drawing. In both, the very best instruction is wasted on those who have no talent for them. It is only the more talented child who will benefit by good instruction and will be able to free himself from the ' shackles of the schema.'

(c). *Exceptional talents.* Unless we are labouring under a delusion, there seem to us to be some children who, from the very outset, are not subject to the schema, or, at any rate, to its most obvious faults. From early childhood their drawing is effortless and realistic, although they have never had any instruction. I am thinking, in this connection, of a special group of so-called ' wonder children ', not of those who have a remarkable talent for copying or lithographing. These children are particularly fond of making copies of heads and the like, (lion, human, etc.) from pictures, and later even from life. They can reproduce them to the minutest detail, but without the least expression, and they fail in the simplest task to be done from memory or imagination. Such achievements are certainly remarkable, but can not properly be called drawing. At any rate they are not organically developed from the drawings which the child does from memory. The most interesting psychological problem is presented by those talented children who draw entirely from memory. The horses represented in Plate III, were drawn by a boy eight years of age, whom Kerschensteiner discovered. The boy drew them and fifteen similar sketches in the presence of his teacher in

PLATE III

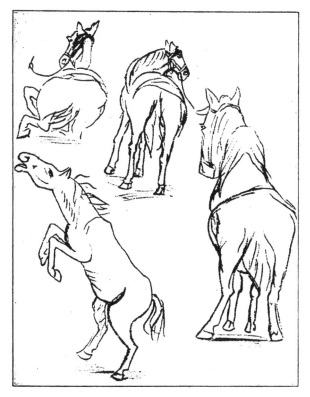

MEMORY DRAWINGS OF AN EIGHT YEAR OLD BOY.
(From *Kerschensteiner* Two-thirds natural size.)

a very short time. "The boy had mastered every expression of activity in a horse with complete certainty, even if he still made some mistakes in drawing. He wrote them down as it were, just as someone else would write down letters" (Kerschensteiner, p. 136). No doubt routine played a part; but the essential aspects must have continually been taken by the boy from his memory or his imaginative picture of the horse while he was drawing them. And these images had concrete, not conceptual errors. The boy drew, not from knowledge, but like a true painter from concrete memory images. This, then, is the point at which we can lay a finger on the psychological puzzle of the wonder-child of drawing. The first question to be asked, is whether he was subject to the schema in his early youth, or not. My answer, as I have already indicated, is that he probably was not.

Unheard of achievements by children, which to the lay mind seem miraculous, lose some of their romantic halo and gain much in scientific interest, when Psychology begins to lay the foundation for their explanation. At the age at which such wonder-children are discovered, their first attempts with a pencil have usually been lost to science. I only know of one case in which the drawings of such a child have been kept from the first and published later. This was done by the Breslau drawing master, C. Kik, in the *Zeitschrift für angewandte Psychologie*, 1909. It will be seen that even in the very earliest sketches of this child the worst type of graphical impossibility does not occur. The drawings produced by the children of some primitive peoples would seem to have the same general character. Examine Fig. 10 : these are not the schemata of our children ; they are human beings and animals, in the most divers positions and movements, with proper limbs and real joints, clothed in garments which have been fitted to the bodies.

(*d*). *An analogy from racial Psychology.* Among the primitive peoples of the present day certain tribes of Eskimos, some of the Australian natives, and the bushmen of South Africa produce remarkably realistic drawings. The drawings of the people of the oldest stone age, found in the famous cave dwellings in the south of France, Spain, and the south of Germany, have a similar character (cf. Fig. 11). Although there was considerable progress in

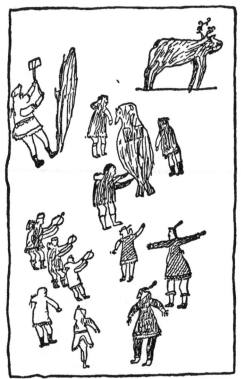

FIG. 10.—DRAWINGS OF AN ESKIMO CHILD.
(After *Maitland*, from *Levinstein*.   Natural size.)

the civilization of the stone age, the art of drawing gradually sank to the level of the schema.   Moreover the bushmen and the Australian natives, who even to-day still draw realistically, belong to the culturally lowest types.   This is a very remarkable fact.   The well-known physiologist and pre-historian, Verworn, has put forward a very bold and original hypothesis to explain this. In his opinion the realistic drawings of these primitive peoples are not to be regarded as the result of long practice and a well-kept tradition, but as the expression of a mind whose original talent for drawing has remained unspoilt. Just as the concept of individual objects, the concrete image, is prior to the abstract concept, so it is the simplest and most natural occupation for the drawing hand to reproduce these individual pictures. Conversely, the schema is evidence of contamination of the spirit. Up

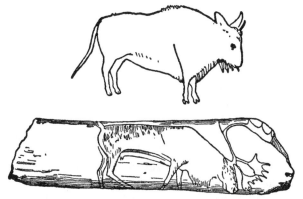

Fig. 11.—Palæolithic Animal Drawings.
(From *Verworn*. The Bison has been reduced.)

to this point I believe his hypothesis to be psychologically correct and it completely agrees with our own interpretation of the drawings of children.

But I cannot quite subscribe to Verworn's conception as to how this reorganization of the mind, which has been so deleterious to the art of drawing, has come about. He puts the blame on the rise of a belief in spirits, that is, animism. When man began to ruminate about death, sickness, dreams etc., and began to believe in the animation by spirits, good or bad, it spoilt his mental life for the purpose of drawing. It seems to me that there are two important arguments against this view. The first is, that our children, whose minds are not filled with animistic conceptions about good or bad spirits, nevertheless draw schematically. The second, a purely psychological one, is that we are dealing not with a reorganization of the *contents* of the mind, but with a *formal* reorganization. It is not at all a question of new contents, new structures of the imagination. Even imaginary things can be drawn realistically, witness the mermaids and dragons of Böcklin, which are as realistic as one could wish. Verworn thinks that mental images must become abstract by the mere process of rubbing up against others when the mind becomes crowded with them. But (happily for our painters) this Herbartian conception of the jostling of images and its mechanical results is psychologically incorrect. As Albrecht Dürer has said, every really great painter is ' inwardly full of pictures.' which do not need to rub off each others corners like the stones in a stream. No, as we shall show later, other factors are involved in the formation of concepts, which is what we are concerned with here. We must once more conclude : it is in the main language which is responsible for the formation of concepts and therefore for the reorganization of mental life and the dominance of conceptual knowledge over concrete images.

This enables us to put forward questions which can be solved empirically. What is the language of bushmen, Eskimos and Australasians like ? Why is it that language has no influence on the drawings of wonder-children ?

REFERENCES :

1. On youthful talents for drawing, comprehensive material is to be found in KERSCHENSTEINER. Three interesting cases are given in Vol. I of *Kind und Kunst,* four more, as well as the first connected treatment of the essay by C. KIK, " Die übernormale Zeichenbegabung," *Zeitschr. f. angew. Psy.* 1909. The interpretations which have only been sketched above, will be found developed in greater detail in my book, *Die geistige Entwicklung des Kindes.*

2. Cave drawings of the stone age and the drawings of primitive peoples : R. ANDREE, " Das Zeichnen bei den Naturvölkern " *Mitteil. d. Anthropolog. Gesellschaft in Wien,* XVII, 1887, p. 100. M. VERWORN, *Zur Psychologie der primitiven Kunst,* 1907, 2nd edn. 1917. *Die Anfänge der Kunst,* 1909. *Ideoplastische Kunst,* 1914.

3. For investigations concerning the attitude of the child towards concrete material other than that at its disposal in drawing, cf. Ch. Bühler, *Kindheit und Jugend*, Leipzig, 1928, p. 102 *et seq.* and p. 166 *et seq.* (on building, and games involving technical construction). V. Neubauer, " Die Entwicklung der technischen Begabung," *Zeitschr. f. angew. Psych.* 29, 1929 (games involving technical construction). M. Bergemann-Könnitzer, " Das plastische Gestalten des Kleinkindes," *Zeitschr. f. Angew. Psych.* 1928. H. Hetzer, " Die Symbolische Darstellung in der frühen Kindheit," *Wiener Arb. z. pädag. Psych.* III, 1926. (Building and drawing.)

CHAPTER SIX

THE EVOLUTION OF THINKING

16.—THE FIRST JUDGMENTS AND THE DEVELOP-
MENT OF THE SENTENCE

(*a*). *The first judgments.* The judgment is the central
core of all human thinking. What is a judgment?
One traditional answer, which goes back to Aristotle, is
that judgments are combinations of concepts.[1] That is
about as correct and as valuable as saying 'a house' is
a combination of stones. Any builder will answer that,
first, there are houses which are not made of stone, and
secondly, not all combinations of stones are houses.
A more modern theory, which is still being worked out,
is connected with the names Hume, Brentano, Stumpf,
Meinong, Husserl and B. Erdmann. This seeks the
explanation as to the nature of the judgment elsewhere.
First, the difference between a judgment and a conception
is that its object is a *relation* and not anything individual.
Or, expressed differently, the subject matter of a judgment
is formulated in language by a 'that'-sentence: that
twice two makes four, that God exists, that there is
thunder, that there is historical justice, or, as we might
say in general, 'that this or that is the case.' It is
always this kind of statement with which judgments
are concerned.

Secondly, in the act of judgment we take up an
attitude towards the subject matter. The specific

[1] It is worth noting that there is another very apt definition in
Aristotle according to which a judgment is *A Statement that may be
true or false.* This is probably the best definition for the purposes
of logic. It would be beyond the scope of this book to show in what
way it agrees with our psychological analysis.

character of this attitude is conviction, *certainty*. If I merely repeat a sentence after someone, without inner participation and without conviction, I am not making a judgment. Certainty has many degrees, from mere suspicion to unshakable conviction which nothing can alter. In the judgment this certainty refers to the relationships existing within the subject matter and can, indeed, refer to nothing else. For although I can say, " I am convinced of the faithfulness of a friend," or " I am certain of a legacy," this is merely an abbreviation for ' that '-constructions, (that a friend is faithful, that I shall receive a legacy).

Thirdly, certainty is based on *reasons*. There are, of course, blind, unreasonable convictions as well, for instance in dreams and as a result of suggestion. The mass-suggestion of politics and the authoritative suggestion of teachers often lead to blind convictions. But these need not concern us here. True conviction must be open-eyed and must have reasons. I repeat : we understand a relation and take up an attitude towards it in which conviction (certainty) is the determining principle and we base the conviction on criteria (reasons) by means of one and the same mental function. Cogitation and doubt (which so often precede conviction) also belong here ; cogitation is partly the seeking after reasons, doubting is the vacillation of conviction. The question now arises as to how this whole complex of functions grows in the mind of the child, and where and when it can be first observed. A child of six months gives as yet no indications ; the two-year-old judges. Therefore all these activities which go to make up the function of judging, must have arisen in that time.

We do not as yet know how this development began, but we know more or less where to look for its beginnings. I shall cite two examples. The first is an observation made by W. Stern. The photograph of its nurse was shown to a child aged 1 ; 4. First it said ' auntie,' but then hesitated, looked at the nurse who was standing near, again at the picture, once more at the girl, and at last joyfully exclaimed " betta ! " (i.e., Bertha, the name of the girl). What was happening here ? First the reaction with a familiar word ; in the end a more specialized interpretation ; in between, hesitancy, looking to and fro, and finally the joyful solution. If we could affirm that the hesitation expresses a doubt, then we should also be correct in attributing certainty to the solution. If the alternate examination of picture and nurse had the value of a comparison, then we could assume that the child finally apprehended the similarity between the picture and the girl, that is, *it apprehended a relationship*. As the second example I give an observation made by Preyer during the 23rd month. " The child took the cup in both hands and drank. The milk was too hot for him, so he quickly put the cup down and, looking at me with wide-open eyes, said in a loud and determined voice, with intense seriousness : *hot*." " In the same week the child went to the oven, stood in front of it, looked at it carefully and suddenly said with great determination : *hot*."

Preyer claims that these are the first judgments which his child formulated in language, and I do not doubt that they were real judgments. But if science is to advance, it must look for objective criteria. What tells us that these were judgments ? We must construct a doctrine of criteria. If judgments are a new acquisition of the mind, they must be distinguished in some recognizable way, by *the manner in which they are brought about*, or by their *attendant phenomena*, or by their *effects*. If we examine the story about the cup of milk, we find nothing distinctive, either in the way in which the reaction occurs, or in its effects, for a cat placed in front of hot porridge behaves in principle in exactly the same way, except that she does not say *hot*. In so far as this is naming, it certainly transcends the capabilities of the cat. But not every pronouncing of a name is judgment. The points of distinction are therefore to be sought only in the accompanying phenomena, the gestures and the modulation of the voice. That the child looks up at the father, is not remarkable, when merely taken by itself, for even a dog will look up at its master in a similar situation, as though 'seeking help.' That is the 're-leasing function' of gestures. Nor is opening the eyes wide a special criterion. In small children it is merely a sign of attention, which can be observed a few weeks after birth. So there only remains, 'loud and determined speaking.' This is the adult's method of accentuating his expressed conviction. If he speaks the sentence, "there is a God!" clearly, decisively and in a certain tone of voice, he underlines, as it were, his expressed conviction. Often an expressive bodily mimicry is resorted to, the body is stiffened, and the fist or foot is used as an organ of expression. We speak of 'taking up an attitude,' of a 'standpoint.' The original meaning of these expressions is probably to take up a position and make preparations for defending oneself. How do matters stand in the case of the child? If we wish to clear up our notions as to how the first experiences of conviction arise, these things will have to be carefully investigated.

Finally, we spoke of the effects of judging. Let the reader imagine as vividly as he can, and with all the gruesome details, that the building he is in at the moment is on fire. This will probably leave very little effect on his practical attitude. The faintest suspicion, however, that the house is really on fire, would have quite different consequences, without the need for vivid imagination. The adult is guided, within wide limits, by his convictions and not by his imagination. At what point in early childhood does this begin? Let us assume that the experience with the oven, which Preyer relates, occurred in late autumn, when the oven is sometimes lit and sometimes not, and that the little man ($1\frac{1}{2}$-$2\frac{1}{2}$ years of age) has already discovered the truth of the proverb about the child who has burnt his fingers, even if only by means of a hot cup of milk. He now goes up to the *cold* oven. He obviously wants to touch it, but hesitates. He does not as yet know the method of carefully and gradually bringing the hand closer. To touch the oven means taking a risk. It is possible that chance brings about the decision, by giving the victory to one side or another in the struggle of motives. But we can imagine a completely different solution, namely, that a conviction is formed through the coming into play of criteria. The bright or dark door of the oven, or, later, some memory of the child may provide starting points. When the child takes the risk *on the basis of such criteria*, then we have found the new function in its mind for which we have been seeking. We are face to face with a conviction based on reasons. Careful observations of this kind of behaviour will be of great service to science. I am inclined to believe that particularly favourable conditions for investigating would be presented by some older, mentally backward, child.

(*b*). *The development of the indicative statement.* Not every proposition which looks like a judgment, contains one. Modern logicians (Riehl, von Kries, B. Erdmann, Külpe) are beginning to separate propositions expressing judgments, from those which subserve a true naming function. If I give a new name to a new object, or allocate arbitrary letters to the corners of a triangle, the sentence which expresses this does not make the same kind of statement as, for instance, the sentence ' The oven is hot.' For definitive sentences of that type do not express the fact that something is, but indicate what ought to be. Besides these ' creative ' definitions there are also ' re-creating' definitions, which determine what a word means according to the common usage of speech : ' N. is called . . .,' or ' N. means . . .' this or that. These are true representations of fact, whose general context is simply ' meaning,' i.e., it establishes between the name and its meaning a relation that has been deduced from the common usage of the word, or from some system, e.g., of scientific terms. Finally, there are sentences which are not naming sentences, although they look like them. When we read in the Bible "his name is Israel, for he strove with God," the qualifying clause merely tells us that the name indicates his nature. It therefore contains a statement of fact, nothing else, just like those sentences of recognition or classification, as when the police examines a man and says 'That is N.N.' or the jeweller says, of a stone, 'That is a diamond.'

What is the objective meaning underlying the names given by a child to objects? We have already noticed that the child behaves as though it had discovered the general truth that every object has a name. I hope no one will venture to make the trivial remark that a child one year of age can not be credited with such profound philosophical penetration! Naturally not in the way in which we have formulated it. What is at the bottom of the ' as though ' is at present an insoluble problem ; but on it depends the further one, whether the simple acts of naming, which the child henceforth carries out with such obvious pleasure, can be called judgments or not. It certainly is a fact that the simple finding of a name, when we adults wish to express something, runs its course without the ponderous apparatus of conviction, insight and reasoning. It is merely a case of an association springing into being at the right instant, followed by a reproduction of the suitable words. Similarly it is probable that in the case of the simple acts of naming of the child, which proceed without difficulty, the sight of the object releases the articulation of a suitable name. It is only those exceptional cases which do not run smoothly that provide an opportunity for hesitation, attentive scrutiny, or looking from one to the other, so that the final solution is arrived at with conviction. In other words, they turn the giving of a name into an act of judgment.

Whatever the explanation may be, it is at any rate certain that at this stage the child expresses everything that is on its mind by means of single words. Since every such word is a linguistic achievement, complete in itself, the apt term *one-word sentence*, has been introduced. It would be very far off the mark to think that all one-word sentences must be either word-reproductions or judgments.   When the child lovingly caresses its doll and calls it ' good,' or when its whole face lights up on seeing something brown which it calls ' chocolate '; when with angry tears it calls the chair ' naughty ' or with wide-open eyes it seeks shelter behind its mother and denounces that threatening, strange being as ' man,' its primary concern is by no means that the thing should receive its right name, or any name.   Quite different attitudes than the one we call judgment, appear and are expressed as well.   But we lack as yet the scientific methods for classifying these things theoretically, distinguishing them by means of objective criteria and following the development of each one separately.   I suspect that a very wide variety of sentences is present here in embryo.   But they will all be found to be concerned with indication, release and representation in close interconnection.   In the end, however—whether from inner causes, or because it is like that in the language of adults—the representational function becomes the dominant one and all the other functions are subordinated to it.

What is the poet's method, when he wishes to express *Stimmung*, a mood or ' atmosphere,' by means of words ? He places one representational sentence next to the other :

> *Über allen Wipfeln ist Ruh*
> *In allen Gipfeln spürest Du*
> *Kaum einen Hauch——*

(Peace broods over the wood, in all its crowns hardly a breath is stirring).

He relies on the music of his words, on his method of representing certain facts about the picture in his mind, to reproduce the ' atmosphere.'   He cannot proceed like the musician, since words that are not names, or word forms that are not part of the representational function, are far too rare and have been neglected too much by language. That is what we mean, when we speak of the dominance of the representational function. But who would deny that, theoretically, matters might be different?

In a chapter on thinking it is obvious that above all the development of the representational sentence must be considered. For several months, up to a year, after the child has learnt to talk sense, all its linguistic requirements are satisfied by one-word sentences. That these are effective is due in the first place to the simplicity of the requirements themselves; they vary very little and are usually so closely bound up with the present perceptual situation, that they can be guessed by the adults without much difficulty. The oral expression is supported by modulations of the voice, in which excitement, calm, nervous tension, desire, satisfaction, pleasure, pain, etc., are easily distinguishable, and by gestures which indicate striving or repulsion and various emotions. Nevertheless, it is usually difficult to understand a strange child completely. One can only find out what it is aiming at, or what actions will satisfy its desires, after one has associated with the child for some time. But apart from that, parents usually attribute far too much logical sense to the words of the child.

On the whole, this will not have any bad results, unless the parents enter too slavishly into the imperfections of the child's language, or by continual and serious misunderstanding, tend to hamper its progress. Until the development from the one-word, to the *two and more-word sentence* takes place from within, the child has no desire to leave his one-word sentences, nor can he be trained in any way to speak two of his childish words together. The time at which this development takes place, usually lies round about the second half of the second year, in children who have received good mental training. I have found one case where it occurred as early as the 14th month and also know of cases where it came late in the third year, but we cannot draw far-reaching conclusions from this, either in a favourable or an unfavourable sense. What does this progress towards sentences containing more than one word signify ? The explanation which lies to hand would be, that there is an improvement in the ability to speak, so that the inner preparation for speaking several words simultaneously can proceed in the organs of speech. We could draw an analogy from playing the piano : the beginner has to play each note separately, whereas the more advanced student can grasp a long succession at once and translate it into co-ordinated finger movements. Besides this improvement in the ability to speak, the sentence of more than one word presupposes that one and the same motive for speaking can give a large number of stimuli, which produce many words. Finally, when each one of a number of words expresses a part, or some aspect of the total meaning, a certain organization begins to show itself in the thought of the child. According to Wundt, in the genesis of a sentence its general unitary sense is present before any organized articulation takes place. It seems that this is the case in adults, and therefore it will probably be the same in the child. It is true that the first sentences which contain more than one word do not, as a rule, give much indication of this. Many of them are nothing more than *twin sentences of one word*, containing two exclamations like, *mama, papa !* or two names like *auntie Betty*, in one breath. But now the transition from two to more words presents no great difficulty and soon crowds of words are strung together without any apparent order, as in the sentence : *fallen tul bein anna ans*, which, transcribed into normal German, would read : *Hans* (who is telling this) *ist ans Bein von Annas Stuhl gefallen.* (Hans has fallen against the leg of Anne's chair).

Cl. and W. Stern have rendered a great service in their book on the language of the child, by collecting all the sentences of two or more words that were known at that time and had come from reliable observations, and attempting to find their structural principles. All the problems involved have not as yet been solved. I think it would be well worth while for a philologist with a psychological training to take up these problems afresh, on a larger scale and with more modern methods. Above all, rhythm, speed and the melody of language will have to be carefully investigated. We do not as yet know anything about the way in which these important methods of expression are acquired and used by the child, or how it uses them syntactically in building up a sentence. They are most likely to appear in a pure form and to be most important before the appearance of conjugation, declination and other kinds of syntactic modifications of words. Something is at least intelligible and known about the structure of primitive sentences, e.g., antithetic order, which is much favoured. This is evident in sentences in which something is first affirmed, after which its opposite is once more specially negated : *stul nei nei—schossel=chair no no—lap*=I don't want to be in the chair, but in your lap ; *gosse nich puppe holn, kleine ja=large not doll fetch, small yes*=I don't want to fetch the large doll, but the small one ; *ollol pa nä, ich pa ja=ollol some no, I some yes*=not Rudolf, but I must be given some (chocolates)

(c). *The inflection of words.* At first all words used by the child are non-inflected units, or if you will, formless. That is, in whatever connection they are used, they always appear in the form in which they were originally assimilated by the child, substantives in the nominative case, verbs as infinitives, adjectives in the positive form and without case-endings. They are all names for something and at the same time serve to indicate a wish or release some action. We can only guess which one of these basic functions is the most important one in any particular case, by taking into account the tone of voice, the gestures and the general situation. Comparative philology ought to give special attention to this form of language. If my observations are correct, exclamations, commands and calls (vocatives), are the first to become more rigid, conventionalized, so that we may look upon these as the first forms. It must be well understood, however, that they are not phonetic forms, but *forms of meaning*, which are accompanied by certain recognizable modifications in the pitch and intensity of the voice (melody and rhythm). The phonetic forms which are the basis of such modulations do not influence each other even when they are placed next to each other in sentences, (*daddy good; Jack naughty*). The naïve listener unthinkingly interprets such groups of words in terms of his own developed sense of language, which demands subject and predicate in a sentence and expects that names, adjectives and adverbs should appear in it in a certain order. But we do not know how the child thinks in this respect. It would be worth while, using psychological and philological methods, to determine whether objective indications can be found of the way in which the various types of words develop in the mind of the child from the general naming function, and in accordance with the increasing need for expression of the child's advancing capacity to think.

For several months, up to a year or even more after it begins to speak, the child does not inflect its words. With German children the beginning of inflection occurs about the beginning of the third year. But, as we have mentioned before, there are wide individual differences. I have seen it occur at 1 ; 3 in the child that formed sentences containing more than one word as early as 1 ; 2 (cf. p. 134). At 1 ; 5 this child was actually capable of spontaneous word transformations. The formless stage will probably always co-exist for several months with the one-word or more-word sentences. Then the chief inflections of words, declination, conjugation and comparison, all appear at about the same time, a proof that they are probably all due to the same mental advance. Imitation runs ahead of creation, and so at this stage the child is simply a small, somewhat abbreviating and mutilating, echo. It hears *nun wird spazieren gegangen* and automatically affirms *baz egangen ;* it hears *gehen wir* and says *gehen wir.* Sometimes it hears *gross* and sometimes *grösser.* It repeats the words and henceforth these two forms are incorporated into its vocabulary, although we cannot as yet say whether the child knows that they belong together. This soon changes. We have a certain sign that a change is taking place, namely, the *formation of analogies.* As soon as a number of forms of the same kind have been learnt, like *grösser, länger, stärker,* a dozen others appear, among them some which do not occur in the language of adults, like *güter* instead of *besser, vieler* for *mehr, hocher* for *höher,* from *es ist nacht* is derived *es ist noch nächter.* These forms must have been invented by the child after the pattern of others, like *gut–güter* after *gross—grösser,* which shows that it has understood the relation between them, and that these forms belong together in the child's mind.

The independent creation of words by the child itself is most clearly evident from these *false* creations. But it would be an unwarranted assumption to think that they are only produced in this way. On the contrary, in the majority of cases the correct form will appear in these analogies. From the astonishingly large number of false and unusual forms which are invented, we may conclude that the principle of analogy is particularly active in the mind of the child and that there is a constant readiness to create new forms after the pattern of the old, or rather with the help of the old. But in what way the old forms help is not known to Psychology. Cl. and W. Stern go so far as to assume that, *after the child has accepted a relatively small number of forms, it acquires the large number of other forms by its own efforts.*

We shall have occasion for a more detailed consideration of the principle of analogy in the thought of the child, when we analyse the processes of deduction. Let us first glance at the well-known and obviously false forms collected in Stern's book. We see from them that

German children simplify matters by using the so-called weak conjugation for all verbs, so that forms like *gebleibt, geesst, getrinkt, gegiesst, genehmt* are used (instead of *geblieben, gegessen . . . genommen*). They sometimes treat nouns like adjectives : *es ist nächter, es ist nog tager* (it is nighter, it is more dayer). But the inventive genius of the child is nowhere more apparent than in its *word combinations and derivations : mama-bah* and *ilda-bah* (old and young sheep, Hilda being the child's own name) ; wakingshirt (*Wachhemdchen*) as opposed to the shirt worn at night[1] ; *eissheiss, bitterheiss, wanderheiss ; mausetrocken ; hintermorgen, übergestern ; einblättern ; hinaufgeliebt.* Typical derivations are : *eine nasserei ; besuppt ; vollgeascht ; benacken ; lebendigen ; der mappler; hergeblasen.*[2]

The fact that disturbances of the process of development may retard the formation of words, is interesting theoretically. There are children who show no serious defects in intelligence and yet at the age of five are incapable of forming grammatically correct sentences themselves, or speaking them correctly after someone else. Their speaking consists of words which are strung together without inflections (*agrammatismus infantilis*). In less pronounced cases we find the beginnings of inflection, with characteristic, serious mistakes ; sometimes only the finer rules of synthesis give difficulty to older children, so that at the age of twelve they still speak like

---

[1] An approximate rendering of the following words into English would be : icehot, bitterhot, wonderhot ; mouse-dry ; after-morrow, over-yesterday ; to leave into (the child was collecting leaves into a paper bag) ; loved up (the child had climbed on to its father's lap and had caressed him) ; a wet mess (where water had been spilt) ; souped (of the spoon with which soup had been eaten) ; ashed (thrown full of ash) ; nakeden (to make naked) ; bring-to-life ; the bagman (a messenger who was carrying a bag) ; blown along (the soldiers with a band in front came " blowing along.")

[2] Only a few particularly remarkable forms have been selected from the rich material. We should have a wrong impression if we expected all of them and only these from every child. By far the greatest number is clumsy and without æsthetic charm. We cannot assume that the naïve child feels this in the slightest degree. Nevertheless, if the adult creator of language (e.g., the poet) wants to find his colleagues, he must go to the child.

foreigners who laboriously have to build sentences out of a large vocabulary. This class of impediment probably results from lack of practice due to other, more primary impediments such as stuttering or stammering. Where such, more external causes could not be found, defects of attention and memory have been held responsible. But it seems to me that we can reach a more accurate determination of the causes by comparing these deficiencies with analogous ones remaining in previously normal adults after a stroke or other injury to the brain. The *finding of words* can proceed almost without a mistake, while the grammatical *formation of sentences and inflection of words* have been seriously impaired. Two processes are, therefore, involved and within certain limits these are independent of one another. A more accurate investigation of these relations in the case of the child would be of the greatest importance to the Psychology of Language.[1]

The principle of analogy is a method, a tool in the mind of the child. What are the purposes of language, the needs of language, which this tool serves and to which it owes its development ?

Let us take as an example the comparison of adjectives. For some time, the child is accustomed to say and think *daddy big, dolly small*, and it soon begins to place these sentences next to each other with so much emphasis, that it is clear he is not merely concerned with each assertion by itself, but also with the relation between them. This relation will first be one of simple opposition, just as the child expresses its emphatic *yes* and *no* in the antithetic ' more-word sentences ' (cf. p. 134). Later it will be differentiated into the relation more–less of size. Even this could in some cases be expressed by using already familiar methods, e.g., by repetition, accentuating

---

[1] A. Liebmann, "Agrammatismus infantilis." *Arch. f. Psychiatrie* XXXIV. 1901. E. Villiger, *Sprachentwicklungen und Sprachstörungen.* 1911. A. Pick, "Die agrammatischen Sprachstörungen," 1. Teil. *Monograph. aus. dem Gesamtgebiet d. Neurologie und Psychiatrie,* VII Heft. 1913. Fröschels, *Psychologie der Sprache,* 1925.

the adjective or employing special words like *more* and
less. A careful examination will show that there is
evidence for this assumption. And now imitation, at
first no doubt only thoughtless repetition, begins to
introduce the new method of expressing the modifications
of words, which in our case is the formation of the comparative. Once again we are confronted with one of the
great, far-reaching discoveries in the history of the
development of language in the child. Just as the child
understands that everything has a name, so he sooner
or later discovers the basic principle of all inflected
languages, that relations can be expressed by changing
the form and the sound of words. He makes this discovery when he stands, as it were, with one foot already
in the mechanics of transformation. Nothing is more
characteristic of true discovery than generalization, the
application of a principle which has been grasped, to the
most varied fields in which it is valid. We should,
therefore, be obliged to predict in theory what is already
evident in practice, that the principal forms of inflection
should appear simultaneously in the child.

(*d*). *The structure of the sentence.* As scientists, we
hardly know more about the finer structural relationships
within a sentence and the development of its framework
than is immediately obvious to any observer. Sentence
is strung next to sentence, and as conjunctions are as yet
almost completely absent, the impression of mere juxta-
position is produced. Whether what follows is an ex-
tension, a closer definition, limitation, condition, exposition or anything else, has to be guessed from the content,
the situation and the modulation of the voice. The
beginning of subordinate sentences marks a big advance,
not only of speaking, but of thinking. The children
observed up to now, who had been brought up in cultured
surroundings, made this advance generally before the end
of their third year. In one case I have observed the use
of the whole system of German subordinate sentences
fully a year earlier. In general the temporal and relative

clauses, which express relations of a more external kind, and indirect questions, which are of great importance to the child, are likely to come first ; causal, conditional and final subordinate clauses last. Irrational conditional clauses, according to Stern's observations, present the most difficulties.

REFERENCES :

Little work had been done in the theory of the development of judgment in child psychology before the present attempt. Most noteworthy are the ideas of K. Groos and W. Stern on the subject in the books mentioned on p. 34.   On the development of the sentence, cf. CL. and W. STERN, *Die Kindersprache*. My own conception has been more fully worked out in *Die geistige Entwicklung des Kindes*. The implications for the theory of the sentence to be drawn from the distinction between the functions of indication, release and representation have been traced in the following essays :   K. BÜHLER, " Kritische Durchmusterung der neueren Theorien des Satzes," *Indogerm. Jahrbuch,* VI (1919) :   " Vom Wesen der Syntax," *Festschrift f. Karl Vossler, Heidelberg (Winter)* 1922. " Über den Begriff der Sprachlichen Darstellung," *Psychol. Forschung* III (1923), p. 282.

17.—THE DERIVATIONS FROM JUDGMENTS : DEDUCTION AND INFERENCE

The first facts are apprehended by the child through perception. They are, as we have seen, such simple facts as *that the oven is hot, that the doll is asleep*, or *that the parrot is not there* (on his usual stand) (cf. p. 88). In the last example memory plays a clearly recognizable part, but previously acquired knowledge will often be involved even where it is not immediately obvious. By far the greatest number of simple interpretations now made by the child in its sentences about perceptual situations, are repetitions of former observations that it has either made itself, or taken over from other people. When the big task of giving names has been completed and practice at simply naming things is no longer so essential, the child begins to make statements ' that so and so is the case.' W. Stern has distinguished three phases in the early thinking of the child, after the most important words have been acquired—the substantive, action, and relationship phases—because words which denote events and actions occur later than substantives, while the majority of adjectives and relatives occur later still. This is understandable, because words expressing time, qualities, and relations only receive their proper functions in statements.

Among the new judgments of the child, we are particularly interested in those which seem to be derived from others, or, more generally, in all those which come about in some way by the help of others. From theoretical considerations we can predict that in principle this can happen in two ways : either the subject changes while the method, that is, the function of judgment remains the same, or vice versa, the subject remains constant for different conclusions. Unfortunately there is a lack of adequate, sound observations. I shall try to show what I mean by a few examples of a kind that will be familiar to everyone.

(a). *The principle of analogy.* When the child makes two-word sentences that definitely have the character of judgments, it will happen that he is not satisfied with one such achievement (*daddy good*). To keep to this example, he will give every one of those present the same attribute (*mama good, aunty good*, etc.). The stimulus for the second and the following sentences obviously does not come from outside ; the child is simply repeating its first act of judgment with other subjects. He is, as it were, turning about in a circle with his scheme, in order to place in it all the other persons, one after another. Or, to put it another way, he is keeping the method constant and applying it to different cases. I do not know whether at this early age it can also happen that the subject remains constant in the same way, while the predicate is changed because of a desire for variation, or whether it is even possible that S and P change simultaneously, so that we may talk of an almost empty schema of judgment, or, figuratively, of a ' blank schema.'

This sticking to one method and applying it in different

cases, is a principle of the highest theoretical interest. It is nothing else than the most general formula of the *principle of analogy ;* it is a lever not merely for thinking, but for man's imaginative activity as well.[1] New conceptions and ideas are arrived at either by additively combining already known elements—$N = \Sigma$ (a, b, c . . . n) —or by applying a method (M) with which we are familiar, to a single given case—$N = M$ (A). Thus the dwarf and the giant, for example, are obtained by making a man larger or smaller, according to our second formula, and in this way, too, new judgments are formed by substituting a new object in the familiar schema. How great the influence of analogy is in the mind of the young child, we have seen above in our discussion of the formation of words. I have no doubt that closer examination would bring to light a wealth of varieties of analogical derivations from judgments. And not only in the child ! When Aristotle attacks a problem, we can predict with fair certainty that he will end by dividing it into matter and form, in Hegel everything is ordered according to a threefold evolution and lesser spirits all have their lesser methods.

In our first example thinking was intimately connected with speaking, therefore we could look upon either the thought schema or the sentence schema as the one that is kept unaltered. It has rightly been said that language thinks for us. If we wish to fathom psychologically the meaning and the far-reaching consequences of this statement, we should have to start from the young child and pay equal attention to both the analogical and the combinatory achievements which we owe to language.

(b). *Inferences with regard to objects.* Thought gives to the isolated objects of perception a connection of being and happening. They are ordered, receive meaning, a past and future. The lasting result of this ordering process will be given in the next paragraph. In a systematic

---

[1] Cf. W. Stern, *Die Analogie im volkstümlichen Denken,* 1893, and the book by Ch. Bühler mentioned on p. 105.

treatise this would be the place for discussing the processes of inference that complete and explain objects, if we knew anything about them. There is an interesting and important phase of development in which the desire to think further along a certain line expresses itself in a very characteristic way. That is the *period of repeatedly asking why*, which in bright and well brought up children usually begins about the end of the third, or at the beginning of the fourth year and lasts for many months. Every teacher knows these questions. But he regards them chiefly as of pedagogical interest for the future, and that is why we know so very little about the state of mind out of which they arise. Sully gives, as usual, a brilliant description : "The fact that the questioning follows on the heels of the reasoning impulse might tell us that it is connected with the throes which the young understanding has to endure in its first collision with a tough and baffling world."[1]

If I am not mistaken, the first desire for explanations grows out of the simple statements of fact which the child makes. Before me stands a girl, $2\frac{1}{4}$ years old, who has just passed out of the phase of stating simple facts and characteristics. What the child has lately been demanding of us, is to be told short stories in which some relation of dependence is expressed, e.g., at table the story of "*Suppen Kaspar*." The child shows us with her hands how thin Kaspar is, but beyond that she probably understands precious little of the story. What the father and the mother say to him has to be repeated word for word and with due emphasis over and over again, and the little listener acts for us Kaspar's aversion to eating soup. But here the tale has begun to merge into perceptual reality. Only the relation of dependence is productive in her thought : "When N. (the child's name) eats soup, then she can push the cart, when N. is big, then . . . when N. is good, then . . ." etc. These sentences containing 'then' are now the favourite

[1] *Studies of Childhood,* 2nd edn., p. 75.

schema for her games of thought and fancy. Only rarely, and as it were accidentally, does she produce anything original. The sentences nearly always have the same contents and are only completed when there is some perfectly familiar association connecting the two parts. Sometimes she begins to speak a 'when' sentence in a beautifully melodious voice, but when she gets as far as 'then,' she sticks, with half-open mouth, wide eyes and a characteristic posture of the head. She has come to the end of her resources and there must be a yawning emptiness in her consciousness. We can see quite clearly that the relation of dependence exists and works in her mind in a form that is quite vague and is the same (or similar) for all cases. But the child is still far from the age of 'why?' and we cannot as yet speak of a desire for explanation. Would that someone could shed some light for us on the path of development from the one form to the other !

Sully has correctly observed that the first 'why' questions concern that which is new—an observation which Stern has also made—and the questioner is satisfied by some reference to the old, familiar things, even if he is merely told "it has always been like that." "When the sorely tried nurse answers the child's question, *why is the pavement hard?* by saying, *because pavement is always hard*, the accusation of old wives' logic is not as justified as we often think it is." Indeed, among everyday things the urge to ask questions dries up. Hum-drum existence stops even primitive impulses to go on thinking, as we see in the parallel case of the practical thinking of the adult. As far as it is feasible, we can look upon this whole attitude as helping to shorten the otherwise long road to associative habituation towards new things.

A more exact classification will probably disclose variants even in this very elementary type of explanation, and above all different valuations. For instance, there is a great difference between merely giving the new thing an old name and bringing it under some rule,

L

and there are many stages between a rule which merely formulates a present habit, and a logically useful law. I can think of hardly anything more attractive than attempting to distinguish these stages and then tracing them as they arise in the child. But for that reliable methods would first have to be invented. In the meantime we shall have to be satisfied with what our sparse observational material teaches us. The first relations which a child must learn to understand, are those which obtain in the purposive actions of adults, on which the child's well-being depends And in practice the first laws the child comes in contact with are the rules and regulations which govern the actions of adults. When the child therefore comes up against laws of nature within this system of actions, it uses the purposive schema to explain them in the same way. We shall touch on this again in the next paragraph.

REFERENCES:

On deductive thinking in adults. G. Störring, " Experimentelle Untersuchungen über einfache Schlussprozesse," *Arch. f. Psychol.* XI, 1908. J. Lindworsky, *Das Schlussfolgernde Denken*, 1916. H. Ormian, "Das schlussfolgernde Denken beim Kind," *Wiener, Arb. z. päd. Psychol.*, Heft 4, 1926.

18.—THE ORIGIN OF CONCEPTS

The concepts of six-year-old school recruits are in a state of chaos, as every teacher knows. Every investigation which has been instituted and published under the general title, " The circle of ideas of the child during its first year at school," has only served to confirm this fact and to throw light on it from different angles. Nevertheless the child of six has already passed through a tremendous mental development. Indeed, rightly understood, this chaos is not a bad sign, but a good one. It is a sign of activity in his thought, a sign, that he has thought about this or that himself and has of his own accord attempted explanations, however elementary. The boy of six is no longer a child passively accepting everything that happens within the limits of his little world ; he is a young explorer who now and then boldly climbs the fence around him to gaze beyond it.   Think for a moment of an old man and an old woman, somewhat limited, but quite content on their lonely farm.   Such people are not bothered by questions and doubts ; they have a view of the world in which everything is perfectly clear, even why the sun shines or storms come.   But in the head of a young student or teacher of 18 to 20 years many things are not clear, there is a wild effervescence of ideas.   At a much lower level, the mind of the child of six is a similar melting pot.   Two, to two and a half years previously, his mind, like that of the old woman's, was perfectly clear.   Then came the restless period of questioning, asking ' why,' and with it, chaos.   But let us trace this development from the beginning.

(a). *The beginnings*.   The child acquires the concepts operative in daily life by learning to understand and use the popular words expressing concepts.   Only rarely are these clarified and defined as they would be at school. To take an example : what is a lever ?   In popular speech, the reader will think of a pole such as is used to move heavy objects.   Some properties are more, some less important ; it can be of wood or iron, long or short, thick or thin.   For dwarfs it will have to be of different dimensions than for giants.   But it will have to possess a certain rigidity appropriate to its dimensions and to the work it is called upon to do.   A willow twig would not be a lever for tree trunks.

We are dealing here with the distinction between *variable* and *constant* factors, or primary and secondary characteristics.   Every woodcutter knows what is necessary for a practical lever, but it was left to Physics to give a clear definition of the concept, by laying down a *single* property : *a lever is any body which can be turned around a fixed axis*.   All psychological questions that deal with concepts can be systematically derived from this fundamental fact, *the formation of invariants*, though not all of them are of equal importance for our present purpose.

Modern logicians and psychologists attribute concepts to the higher vertebrates as well. They point out that a dog, for instance, recognises his master in the most varied disguises and situations, and that he treats every hare as hare, whether it is brown or blue, or even if it is a rabbit. This may prove that a dog forms invariants, but it must be emphasized that these can only be mere rudiments of our concepts, for *names* are as yet entirely lacking. In section 6 we have described in detail how names arise in the child. I wish to recall once more the fact that soon after the naming function has been acquired, there arises in the child an urge to give everything a name: *everything which is present to the senses of the child must receive a name.* If a sufficient number of words were at his disposal, it would be natural for the child to give every object which is apprehended, recognized, and treated as an individual, its own name, so that only proper nouns such as *Socrates*, *Elbe*, and *Dresden* would arise. The philologists in fact assume that proper nouns are among the oldest acquisitions of language. We can observe the truth of this directly in the child, to whom *papa* and *mama* are at first pure proper nouns.

This state of affairs does not continue, and this may partly be due to an external circumstance, namely the lack of words. There is an infinite number of objects in the world, but the number of words in a language is very limited. If everything is to receive a name, therefore, a large number of objects must receive the same one. The basic schema in our mind for the formation of concepts may be written as follows:

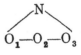

One name stands for many objects (e.g., *dog* for all pugs, whippets, terriers, etc.), and is *associated* with every one of the different conceptions about these objects, and these again are all associated among themselves. But we should be vastly overestimating the influence of external circumstances if we believed that this sufficiently explained the origin of concepts. The forming of concepts must somehow be an expression of fundamental inner laws of the mind itself. In the child we can show that it is promoted and led into definite channels by inner circumstances, which are at first usually looked upon as negative, as defects in the processes aiming at the perfection of mental life. For is it not a defect of accurate perception to confound, as the child does, an apple tree with an oak, or a calf with a large dog ? The rapid fading of memory images may be a factor ; at any rate, in the end it is often not easy to distinguish the effect of such defects from that of thorough abstraction and true abstractions are by no means lacking as the process of giving names runs its course. But there is also a positive witness to the thought which is active in concepts. Could we not suppose that a gradual ascent to higher, i.e., more general and abstract concepts, takes place from proper nouns, that a ' pyramid of concepts ' is built up from them in the mind of the child ? This view is certainly plausible and has been held, but the facts are against it. The building up process takes place simultaneously from above and below, from the concrete and singular as well as from the most abstract and general. Some of the most general concepts, such as *thing, something, do, make, and bring about,* appear unexpectedly early in the thought and vocabulary of the child, a remarkable fact indicating that in this sphere everything does not happen as mechanically as was formerly thought.

(*b*). *The most general concepts (categories).* We have spoken before of the category of a ' thing' with certain properties. We always experience colours, hardness, cold, warmth etc., as properties of something, as properties of objects, and as far as we can see, there seem to be no reasons for thinking that the sense impressions of the child were at one time quite differently constituted from our own. The use of the first words that make sense is somewhat different in the earliest stages of development. Their application is chiefly regulated according to the principle of the constancy of affect and wish, until here, too, the object (*das Ding*) comes to its own and the principle of the *constancy of objects* is established. It is possible that the child first treats names as properties of things, like colours, forms, sizes, hard and soft. One further step has still to be taken. The giving of a name to this principle itself according to which words are used. If we survey the earliest names, we shall as a rule find one or even several that are used, at one time or another, for nearly all the things that catch a child's attention. It may merely be the word *this* or *that*, which is regularly accompanied by demonstrative gestures. It is questionable, however, whether such words accompanying demonstrative gestures always have the function of names, because it is a priori probable that gestures, and even demonstrative gestures, at first only express wishes and affects, just like words. Indeed, this view is supported by observations. Why should the accompanying words be different ? At the same time, it seems worth noting what I have found in the case of a child that was specially observed for this. At the end of 1 ; 7 we noted : " First use of *this* twice running. She sees mother's watch lying on the table and says *want this watch !* Shortly afterwards, she is playing ' cooee ' with a towel (holding towel in front of face and withdrawing it again). Mother takes another towel : *want towel !* exclaims the child. Mother says, ' but you have got a towel.' The child, more emphatically : *want towel !* repeats this several times, till she says with some excitement, stretching out her arm (demonstrative gesture) *want this towel !* On the same day she also said *this pencil*, and *that book*, with demonstrative gestures." The definite name is present in each case, the *that* is probably to be regarded as an accompanying phenomenon to the demonstrative gesture, which would have been adequate without it. Soon, however, *this* and *that* also appear by themselves and are definitely names. At the same time *one* (*ein* or *eins*) appears, before the child has any conception of a number one. It is merely an indefinite name, just as we adults say ' something,' or ' whats-his-name,' or ' *da ist einer,*' some*one* is there. We always had the impression that the particular name did not occur to the child, or that (for some unknown reason) it was of no importance to her. We heard the words *something* and *thing* (*etwas* and *Ding*) much later. More observations will have to be collected on this point. It could be asked whether *that ?   What's that ?* ,are not naming questions and as such contain the generic name for thing. I should not like to assume this, although I have no clearly formulated grounds. I consider the distinguishing feature and the novelty to be only in the meaning of the question and that *that* has no other function than that of a demonstrative gesture.

If we have been on the right track, it would seem that at the stage of giving names, one or other name of an indefinite, universal character arises, sometimes through the use of accompanying gestures. If we ourselves try to define *something*, we can hardly say anything better than that *something* is everything that can receive a name. This is what we meant by the assertion that the category of the thing is a function of thought, or, transferred to the object, that the general property of being namable demands itself a word that is its name. It would be interesting to determine what the conditions are in the most primitive languages.

We now come to the *concept of making*, the category of *causality*. One-sided philosophical empiricism has made many assertions about the origin of the idea of causality in the child, when a careful investigation of facts would have guarded it against insupportable and false theoretical conclusions. It is said, for instance, that the regular sequence of two perceived events, which sets up firm associations, also lays the foundation for the idea of causality. There is some truth in D. Hume's development of this theory. If some preparation, or act, or event that he notices, regularly precedes the meal of an infant, then the well-known expectational reactions of feeding, immediately follow the event. Similar observations can be made in zoological gardens. Perhaps we can even follow Hume a step farther, and assume that in the higher animals and in man, an endless series of such ' experiences ' of itself, i.e., purely according to the laws of associational mechanics, develops the general tendency to keep watch, as it were, forward and backward in time for other events, in other words, to regard every event as a link in a temporal chain, having neighbours on either side. In certain cases a dog actually behaves in a way that would lead one to infer such a general habit of reacting.

Now as this is in no way even thinking, it can still less be the idea of causality, nor did Hume himself assume that it was. But it has been assumed by some of our contemporaries, who regard themselves as his disciples and wish to purge the ideas of the master in order to bring them into accord with pure association psychology. They fail to notice, however, that they are thereby driving the whole spirit out of the theory. In Hume's sense, the reflective thought of man infers or abstracts the idea of causality from that general tendency towards reaction.[1] To avoid misunderstanding, we affirm unconditionally that such a theoretical simplification of the argument is permissible where we are concerned with the problem of the justification of the principle of causality. But it is quite a different matter to assert that this process of abstraction actually takes place in the child and is the final act of the psychological genesis of the idea of causality. Anyone who has ever observed a child, knows that regularly recurring events do not stimulate

---

[1] Put more accurately, only the element of necessity is inferred, which is thought of in conjunction with the causal sequence, while the other elements of the idea of causality have other roots as well. cf. e.g. A. Riehl, *Der philosophische Kritizismus*, Vol. I, 2nd edn., particularly p. 143.

and call forth the child's thought at all. In this respect there is no difference between it and primitive man—or the chimpanzee. The intellect is an instrument for grappling with new, unheard-of situations ; not the rule, but the exception, strangeness, stirs primitive man to think and attempt explanations.

The second error of the purely empiricist theory lies in the assumption that external, physical relations, as in the famous case of the two colliding billiard balls, are the model cases by which the relation of dependence is apprehended. That is certainly not so. Whether chimpanzees have insight or not, we can, at any rate, point to those situations in their behaviour in which insight must arise at some stage of their development, namely, situations where everything depends on apprehending the usefulness of means (tools) in achieving a given end. The first relations that a child grasps, are relations of meaning in a purposive act. The first relations that a child must learn to *understand*, because its welfare depends on them, are those in the purposive acts of adults. The first laws with which it comes into practical contact, are the rules and regulations that govern the behaviour of adults and are meant to govern its own. This presupposes that instinctive ' give and take ' between the minds of a community of living beings, which is called empathy (*Einfühlung*). We have come across this more than once in the course of this book, e.g., on p. 55, in the first words with a meaning that the child understands and imitates, and we have always spoken of the imitation of gestures as the pillars of the bridge from mind to mind. It would be of great value to think out this complicated series of relationships anew from the point of view that interests us here, and to investigate it by empirical methods. For it is here that the key lies to the origin of the idea of causality. It is a fact that at an early age the child ' understands ' natural events that break into the routine of its practical life, according to the schema of a purposive act. Here is an example : The parents, Scupin, made the following note during the 32nd month of their boy : " when we entered the room to-day, the boy stood at the window and scolded, *the sun is very naughty, the sun makes the fingers bloody.* . . . There were finger-marks on the window, from which we concluded that he had held his fingers against the light and had seen the red blood shining through."

What the child at this age has at its disposal for interpreting relations is adequately expressed in the words *make, give, do.* Just as the mother ' makes ' the food and the bed, or ' gives ' the child pleasure, pain, and satisfaction in its many wants and troubles, so the child itself and things in general ' do ' this or that. If I am not mistaken, the general facts outlined for the words make, give, do, are paralleled in the words *that, one, something, thing,* (cf. p. 149, etc.). That is, these words appear remarkably early as general auxiliary words for acts whose names are not known to the child, not at hand or not intended, like "make lalala," (i.e., sing), or, quite generally, the child says, make " so," and demonstrates what it wants done. At 1 ; 5 these were very frequent expressions of my child. I believe the following formulation fits the facts : The category of making or doing, which has probably been active in the thought of the child a long time previously, has attracted to itself a word that expresses it, and that names or describes it where it is intended to interpret external events.

Two further observations may be made before we leave this subject. I have emphasized on p. 136, that the origin of words—their meaning (function), not their form—has still to be investigated psychologically. The specific function of the verb will be connected with empathy and the idea of ' making.' Our basic stock of verbs even to-day still bears the stamp of this childish attitude towards the world. Secondly, when the child treats everything by this method of sympathetic intuition and regards everything that happens as having reference to itself and its needs, we have the beginning of the first systems of philosophy, the purely teleological and egocentric—or, at any rate, anthropocentric—interpretations of nature and life.

(c). *The definitions of the child.* The development of the activity of judgment benefits the concepts, for concepts are junctions in the network of knowledge. (" *Wo ein Tritt tausend Fäden regt. . . . Ein Schlag tausend Verbindungen schlägt* ") : one and the same object appears in different relationships and receives more than one name. We do not need to think only of imaginary names in games of illusion, where a stick is called and used as a horse and many other things ; even in the sober thought about reality the same thing appears under different names : *Elsa, girl, human being, person ;* or *Bello, pug, dog, animal ;* or *hammer, tool, thing.* Here we are confronted with the reversal of a previous observation, that *one* name is given to many things (p. 148). If this interpenetration of the different spheres of names is to mean order and not inextricable chaos, the specific relations of concepts, subordination of species to genus, and co-ordination, must be noticed and respected by the child : that dogs, cats, cows, birds and even fish belong to the animal kingdom, or that the name ' tool ' can be used for hammer and pincers, as well as for all the adjuncts of manual labour. Every teacher knows that this process of ordering the concepts has only just begun when the child enters school, and knows how much the school still has to do. We are interested here in the fact that this process has begun at all, when the child enters school. But let me hasten to add that we do not as yet know how this comes about.

Up to now, only one method has been tried. If we ask a child of four, " what is a spoon, what is a chair ? " the answer will always take the form : " for eating, to sit on " ; or the child will begin to give a long description. " what is an omnibus ? " " For many ladies to sit in. There are soft seats. There are three horses, they run ; one makes " *din* " (the bell is rung), they run " (Binet).

That is the sort of street scene with which Miss five-year-old is acquainted. "What is a snail?" "*C'est pour les écraser, pour pas qu'ils mangent la salade, tout.*" The child is standing in the garden and is making its practical dispositions. "What is a dog?" "He bites, he is held on a chain, he sits up and begs, he runs, he has a tail." Under the influence of the school these definitions according to purpose become rarer. An American investigator (Barnes) has assigned the following percentages to them, starting at the sixth year: 79, 63, 67, 64, 57, 44, 44, 34, 38, 31. Their place is taken by more or less correct definitions, in which logical relations play a part. In former times the child at school learnt to define assiduously according to the well-known logical scheme. This kind of teaching has now been abandoned almost everywhere, and for good reasons: for to demand that the child should at any time be able to recite the genus to which something belongs and the characteristics which define a species, was to overrate considerably the value of purely logical relations. In most fields it is the inter-relationships between things and events as formulated in our laws of nature, which are of greater importance.

Let us return once more to the pre-school age. The dominance of the concept of purpose in the thought of the child is so characteristic, that we may speak of the age in which thought has a *practical orientation towards purpose*. The sphere of things and events of which the child is master in virtue of this category, is certainly not very wide and the network of relations of purpose is not continuous, since it breaks off at every new link. Nevertheless, there are clearness and order in this small domain. That chaos in the minds of 'school recruits,' which practical pedagogues have found, only arises later, through ceaseless questioning, when the child stretches its feelers in every direction into the unknown, when the explanation of purpose has become a useful tool of its thought and a probe boring ever deeper. -

Does the history of mankind show a similar development ? We know how deeply 'animism,' the belief in spirits, stirs the minds of primitive peoples (cf. p. 123). I quote a sentence from Verworn : " The idea that represents the first great attempt at constructing a theory about things, is the gloomy, phantastic, awe-inspiring idea of animating spirits." It is not the task of the psychologist to reconstruct pre-history ; but he is interested in formulating the psychological presuppositions which are contained in our picture of prehistoric times. I believe, that if there ever was a time of paradisean clarity and innocence, it was due to the absence of that restless and boring question, ' why ? ' Man recognized and accepted the obvious practical purposes of nature and of life like the child, without demons and spirits in the background, for the simple reason that a desire for explanation going beyond the circle of things necessary to life had not yet been born.

REFERENCES :

The thinking of the infant: Jean Piaget,'*The Language and Thought of the Child* (International Library of Psychology, 1925). *Judgment and Learning in the Child* (International Library of Psychology, 1927). *The Child's Conception of the World* (International Library of Psychology, 1929). *The Child's Conception of Physical Causality* (International Library of Psychology, 1930).

CHAPTER SEVEN

SOCIAL BEHAVIOUR

19.—CONTACT AND THE UNDERSTANDING OF EXPRESSION

IN the foregoing pages we have shown how the child gradually learns better control over the world around it, after the initial helplessness of the newborn infant. But with the exception of a few facts mentioned in connection with the development of speech, we limited ourselves to the relations of the child to its objective environment. We shall now deal with the contact between the child and the human beings that surround it, and investigate when this contact begins, of what sort it is, and how it becomes more complex in the course of development.

(*a*). *The first stages of social contact.* Man, in his specific characteristics as man, is of almost no importance to the newborn infant. A mother may think that her crying child becomes quiet when she takes it into her arms or speaks soothingly to it, because it somehow feels that another human being is near ; but she is entirely mistaken. It was possible to show experimentally, that the child is also pacified if the bed is lifted up without disturbing it, or by making any sounds whatever. The determining factor is not the presence of someone else, but the change in position or the auditory stimulus.[1] When the child becomes quiet on being given a hot water bottle or a soft cushion, or on being caressed by the mother, we have an exactly similar case. In a similar way we have to interpret the well-known phenomenon of transference of crying in very young siblings, which can

---

[1] H. Hetzer and B. H. Tudor-Hart, " Die frühesten Reaktionen auf die menschliche Stimme." *Quellen u. Studien zur Jugendkunde,* 5, Jena, 1927.

frequently be observed in a home. When one child begins to cry, all its room-mates soon begin too, merely because the crying of another is an unpleasant, disturbing auditory stimulus.[1] In the first few weeks of life, during which all these phenomena can be observed, the child does not distinguish between human beings and other stimuli with which it comes in contact. It is still in the *pre-social* period of its life.

But during the second month a great change takes place. We can already speak here of specific social reactions. The child responds quite differently to a human voice than to any other auditory stimulus. For the sound of a voice is answered by a smile, whilst not even the loveliest sound of a bell will elicit one.[2] That smiling is at first a specific social response and can only be elicited by human beings, is also shown by the reactions of a child to the human face.[3] The child of two to four months only smiles when it sees the face of a person, but not when its attention is directed to colours, shining objects, or a live cat. The first response of the child to persons, as shown in its smile, is therefore positive. The child, which smiles when it sees a face or hears a voice, is *socially responsive*. It can participate in a contact set up by the adult. But it cannot as yet actively set up such a contact itself. Hence there may be a point of social contact between an adult and the child of four months ; but although the child has just been smiling and gurgling at the adult it is incapable of coming into contact with another child of the same age when the two are brought together. They may look at and touch each other, but neither discovers that the other is a human being. Only when their eyes happen to meet, do they sometimes smile at each other.

The child of five or six months, however, is no longer

[1] Ch. Bühler and H. Hetzer, " Das erste Verstehen von Ausdruck im ersten Lebensjahr." *Zeitschr. f. Psych.* 107, 1928.
[2] Hetzer and Tudor-Hart, *loc cit.*
[3] Ch. Bühler, " Die ersten sozialen Verhaltungsweisen des Kindes," *Quellen und Studien zur Jugendkunde*, 5, Jena, 1927.

dependent on such a fortuitous meeting of glances, or on the contact from an adult. It is *socially active* and can, therefore make a contact itself. By cries and touch, it draws the adult's attention to itself. It practically hurls itself on another child of its own age that is brought near. The two children look, smile, and gurgle at each other, touch each other, and soon lively relations are established.

(b). *The first appreciation of expression.* The child of three months, which smiles when it hears someone talking or sees his face, does not observe the facial expression of the adult at all. It will smile if the adult looks friendly, just as it will smile if he looks angry, because at first it merely notices the eye of the adult, and this does not show an angry or friendly expression as much as the rest of the face.[1] Only when the child learns to observe further components of facial expression does it alter its behaviour. The child of five months no longer reacts positively in a single case to an angry face, but answers this stimulus by some negative response. The child of five to seven months simply *reflects* the positive and negative expression of the adult, i.e., it repeats the movements of the adult, such as dropping the corners of the mouth, closing the mouth, pushing the lower lip forward, wrinkling up the forehead when watching an angry face, or opening mouth and eyes wide for a smiling face. Only in the eighth month do these 'reflected' responses make way for a new group, which has up till then not been observed   For instance, the child of eight months turns away from someone who looks angry, and tries to get away from him, but it will come towards a smiling person and hand its toys to him. That is to say, it no longer responds in a simple fashion, but *understands* the other person and the situation. This shows that it now appreciates the other person with respect to the total situation, and his facial movements as determining this situation. The child's behaviour to-

[1] Ch. Bühler and H. Hetzer, *loc cit.*

wards the voice is similar to its behaviour towards the facial expressions. The voice, too, is at first simply a specific stimulus, regardless of tone and elicits a positive response under all circumstances : only at a later stage is a distinction made between scolding and friendly words.

At the end of the first year, the child, which an adult looks at angrily or handles roughly, realizes that this is merely done in play. At first it will reflect the angry expression negatively, like the younger child. Suddenly, however, its unhappy expression will change to a radiant smile. It is beginning to understand that the adult has been merely pretending, and does not mean anything unpleasant.

We may only begin to expect an understanding of gestures, such as threatening to chase the child away, or coaxing it to come closer, when the child has passed the stage of merely 'reflecting' expressions, that is, not earlier than the eighth month. This assumption is borne out by experiment. The eight-months-old answers the threatening or coaxing gestures sensibly. The next step in understanding is now taken by means of language. We may remark in passing that the child of which no one takes any notice and that has not much opportunity of coming into contact with people, remains backward in its capacity to understand expressions even at this age. This defect also shows itself later in the understanding of language and the capacity for self-expression.[1]

20.—THE FORMATION OF GROUPS

(a). *Child and adult.* We saw that the child originally responds positively towards the adult. How far this immediate positive attitude is based on positive experience, which the child has been able to have of adults, or how

---

[1] Hetzer and Reindorf, " Sprachentwicklung und soziales Milieu," *Zeitschr. f. angew. Psych.* 28, 1927 ; and Hetzer, " Kindheit und Armut," *loc. cit.*

far it is based on instinct, cannot be decided here. We shall probably have to admit both possibilities. At this stage the child treats all persons with the same friendliness; no one, not even the mother or the nurse, who are continually active around it, is in any way preferred. Only at the age of nine months and over does it begin to make exceptions. It is friendly with people whom it knows well, but is very shy with strangers, although this shyness towards an unknown visitor can often be overcome in a relatively short time. It cannot be accidental that the child has a different relationship to people with whom it is in constant contact, than to strangers whom it is meeting for the first time, just at the time when it is no longer bluffed by unmotivated scolding, because its relations to adults reach beyond the immediate situation. We are dealing here with a permanent attitude, which is entirely different to the attitude called up by the present situation. People that it knows equally well, are treated with equal friendliness, by the child of a year and a half. *No one amongst them is preferred in any way.* Just as little as we can speak of a preference towards one particular person, can we speak of a hostile attitude towards an adult. It treats him with perfect confidence and it needs him at this stage more than ever before and more than it will need him for a long time afterwards. For at this age the adult has to satisfy all the social needs of the child, since children of its own age play no part at all as playmates, as we shall see. The social demands of the child of one to two years are, however, far higher than those of the sibling, who is satisfied with an occasional smile or a little game played with him by the nurse when she clothed, bathed, or fed him. The child in its second year demands from the adult more than occasional notice. It demands company as such, and company for its games; as soon as it begins to talk, it wants to ask questions, tell stories, receive information.

During the third year a sudden change generally takes place in the relations between adult and child. Agreement and trust are at an end for some time to come. This change is related to the development of the will.[1] Between the ages two and four the child learns to use its will for attaining an end. At first it is, as it were, intoxicated with this new possibility, which it has discovered in itself. We know the little child only too well, which, the whole day long and at every possible opportunity, defiantly repeats ' I want,' answers every other suggestion with an energetic ' no,' and cries or hits and kicks every time its will is thwarted. Ch. Bühler was the first to point out that this period has a positive value for the development of the will, although it is so unpleasant from an educational point of view.[2] On the basis of extensive statistical material about six-year-old children and several years' experience as educational advisers, we can say that if this obstinate, defiant stage is not developed (for reasons as yet unknown), we must expect serious disturbances in the development of the child's will.[3] Children of six and over, who are weak willed and uncontrolled and are in need of constant supervision to keep them at one task, but who, on the other hand, succumb to every temptation, are excessively fond of sweets and cannot bring themselves to do without something, are very often children who have not passed through the ' defiant ' stage.

During the age of ' defiance,' which lasts for several months, the child necessarily comes into conflict with its environment.[4] Up to now it has allowed others to prescribe to it what it wanted ; now it consistently demands the satisfaction of its wishes. The child now follows its own ends ; but it is continually being disturbed by its environment and therefore begins to take up a hostile attitude towards other people. We have to

---

[1] For the development of the will, cf. Ch. Bühler, *Kindheit und Jugend*, loc. cit.

[2] cf. *Das Seelenleben des Jugendlichen*, 5th edn., Jena, 1929.

[3] H. Hetzer, " Entwicklungsbedingte. Erziehungsschwierigkeiten *Zeitschr. f. pädag. Psych.*, 1929,

[4] This crisis of the will has been excellently observed in one case by E. Köhler, *Die Persönlichkeit des dreijährigen Kindes*, Leipzig, 1926.

recognize that it learns to hate people at this age. But it also learns to love them deeply ; for in general the child that turns against its environment attaches itself very strongly to one particular person, from whom it seeks help and protection, and to whom it turns its affection. Its relations with different persons have now become differentiated.

For a short time, but not with respect to every person, a negative social attitude gains the upper hand in the child. As soon as the fact that it can will its own ends ceases to be new, it no longer insists quite so much on having its own way all the time. In fact, we may say that the child of five or six, which has already passed through the crisis of will, is very much inclined to submit to the wish of others. This willingness is connected with the development of a consciousness of task and duty.[1] In place of the pronounced tendency of the three-year-old to do what he wants there is developed a willingness to take over tasks set by others.[2] The child is now exceptionally easy to educate. Only when the child's effort after independence begins to grow again, having its maximum during puberty, are renewed conflicts started between child and adult. The child of six is still easily led ; at nine it begins to revolt ; the youth repudiates being led, and, having set aside the authority imposed on him from without, bows only to that which he has himself chosen.

(b). *The child group.* We have seen that, as soon as the child begins to be socially active, contact between it and companions of the same age begins. Like the adult, the older, socially active child can enter into relations with a younger one, if the latter is already socially active. But the relation between the two children is not one of equality. When two children are brought together, it

---

[1] Cf. Ch. Bühler, *Kindheit und Jugend, loc. cit.*

[2] Cf. Ch. J. Zweigel, " Über die Wirksamkeit von Aufgaben in der frühen Kindheit,' *Wiener Arbeiten zur pädag. Psych.* 5, 1929. Also Ch. Bühler, " Das Sechsjährige in psychologischer Betrachtung," *Handbuch für den Anfangsunterricht,* Wien, 1926.

soon becomes evident whether they are equal and stand
against each other as rivals, or whether one of them has to
play a subordinate rôle.[1] The dominant child, for instance, will grab all the toys and push the other back
roughly if it wants to regain one of the captured objects.
*Before the tenth month the child is hardly conscious of
submission or dominance.* But the child of ten months
already looks around triumphantly, if it has succeeded in
obtaining the rattle after a hard fight, while its vanquished
playmate looks sorrowful.[2] Brute force is, however,
not the only way in which the leader can show his superiority. As early as the end of the first year we find another
kind of leader, who owes his leadership to the circumstance
of his having ' ideas.' If one of the children can do a
number of things with a new toy, while the other had been
at a complete loss, the first will gain the leadership by
drawing attention and admiration to himself. Similarly,
there are even at this age children that take up a sympathetic attitude towards others, consoling them by letting
them have the ball, or helping them in some way, and in
this way achieving dominance.

Although two children one year of age are able to organ-
ize a proper game, alternately giving each other their
toys, or one showing the other how to do something and
the other copying this, *the contact between them is in general
of very short duration.* Soon each of the partners is busy
with himself and his own toys again. The child is only
able to apply itself to its companion to a limited extent,
and its power of persevering is small.[3] Hence the adult,
who applies himself completely to the child and prevents
it from giving up the game too soon, is the real playmate
of the child of one or two. The child of two and over is
capable of playing for a long time, even with other children.

[1] Ch. Bühler, " Soziales Verhalten," etc. *loc. cit.*
[2] Compare the observations on fowls of Schjelderup-Ebbe, "Sozial-
psychologische Beobachtungen am Haushuhn," *Zeitschr. f. Psych.*,
84, 1924.
[3] With regard to the perseverance of young children, cf. H. Beyrl,
" Ausdauer und Konzentration in der frühen Kindheit," *Zeitschr. f.
Psychol.*, 107, 1929.

When several children are playing together, the leadership as a rule rests with the older ones, up to the age of six.[1] But from the schoolgoing age onwards we find that some have the talent for leadership, and from then on we find groups that are led by a child of the same age.[2] That a capacity for leadership is relatively rare among very young children, is shown by the fact that, whenever a larger number of them is present, they prefer to play games with well defined rules. Popular games have many rules, which are strictly adhered to and which determine the action of each individual with great exactitude ; they therefore achieve what the leader would otherwise have to work out in his organization.[3]

Like the ability to lead a group in play, the ability to take part in ever larger groups develops in the course of early childhood. The child of one to two years can only take part in a group of two. It cannot as yet enter into relations with more than one other. At the end of the second year contact is possible between three. The group that contains three or four members is preferred by all young children.[4] The schoolchild, on the other hand, always tries to become a member of as large a group as possible. The greater the rôle of the companion of the same age, the less the importance of adults, to whom the child is in the beginning exclusively attached. The relations between the child and its young companions at first exist side by side with those towards adults, but at length gain the upper hand entirely.

[1] H. Hetzer, " Das Volkstümliche Kinderspiel," *loc. cit.*
[2] K. Reininger, " Das soziale Verhalten von Schulneulingen,"
Wiener Arb. z. päd. Psych. 7, 1929 ; also " Über soziale Verhaltungsweisen in der Vorpubertät, *do.* 12, 1925.
[3] H. Hetzer, " Das Volkstümliche Kinderspiel," *loc. cit.*
[4] S. Wislitzky, " Beobachtungen über das soziale Verhalten im Kindergarten," *Zeitschr. f. Psych.* 107, 1928.

INDEX OF SUBJECTS

INDEX OF AUTHORS